My GLORY
Was I Had
Such
FRIENDS

ALSO BY AMY SILVERSTEIN

Sick Girl

AMY SILVERSTEIN

My GLORY Was I Had Such FRIENDS

A MEMOIR

HARPER WAVE

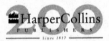

MY GLORY WAS I HAD SUCH FRIENDS. Copyright © 2017 by Amy Silverstein. All rights reserved. Printed in the United States of America. No part of this book may be used or reproduced in any manner whatsoever without written permission except in the case of brief quotations embodied in critical articles and reviews. For information, address HarperCollins Publishers, 195 Broadway, New York, NY 10007.

HarperCollins books may be purchased for educational, business, or sales promotional use. For information, please email the Special Markets Department at SPsales@ harpercollins.com.

FIRST EDITION

Library of Congress Cataloging-in-Publication Data has been applied for.

ISBN 978-0-06-245746-2

17 18 19 20 21   LSC   10 9 8 7 6 5 4 3 2 1

For Scott and Casey

AUTHOR'S NOTE

The conversations in this book are written from my best-efforts recollection and memory to capture the accurate essence, meaning, and sentiment of what was said. All incidents and people are real, although I have changed some names and identifying characteristics to preserve anonymity.

I WANT TO mention here the vital presence and extraordinary role played by my husband, Scott, who was with me in this story every day in every way with infinite heart and mind. And while I could have crafted a beautiful memoir about the glory that was Scott (as I aimed to do in *Sick Girl*), this time around I chose instead to shine a light on women's friendships. Scott has been gracious to support my writing him into the background of this book when, in fact, the inimitable power of his love was front and center in California and was the constant that held each and every one of us afloat while there.

My GLORY
Was l Had
such
FRIENDS

Joy
Jill
Leja
Jody
Lauren
Valerie
Robin
Ann
Jane

We were grown daughters all, some mothers of high school or college kids, a few of us seasoned career women. We had become our middle-aged selves—our wisest, steadiest, most powerful selves yet. And we discovered a new best in ourselves together because I was dying, really dying this time, and we weren't twenty-five anymore.

I had been ill back then too. Shockingly ill. But in our midtwenties, we had not yet become fully formed women. Still emerging into adulthood, we easily turned as moody and flip as self-interested teenagers. Our focus was on dating or setting up newly married lives, finding our way at first jobs or completing graduate school. We floated above small troubles, giggling arm in arm through parties and bars that kept us out late into the New York City night. We invested more in great shoes and best-fit jeans than in how to rise up for a friend who needed some kind of crazy surgery we could not begin to understand.

Our empathy had not ripened at twenty-five.

At fifty, it had.

So in the winter of 2014, when a doctor said that my transplanted heart was in precarious failure, my friends paused their lives and rallied around me. When I was told my best shot at retransplant depended on my husband, Scott, and me moving immediately from our house in New York to a hospital room in California, friends followed in constant rotation—abandoning must-do responsibilities that left husbands scrambling, bosses irritated, and teenagers unsupervised by the crucial mothering eye.

A spreadsheet appeared, and friends signed on for three- or four-day blocks, some for multiple visits, filling every calendar space for March, April, and May so that each woman could pass the baton seamlessly from one to the next. They booked plane reservations for cross-country flights, looking for bargains and counting up frequent-flyer miles, hoping for the best but paying full price if that was what it took to ensure that I would never have to spend a night without one of them there.

When I woke again and again in the darkness of that hospital room so far from home, engulfed by what felt like a literal heart on fire that scorched a line of breath-stopping pain from shoulder to shoulder, my friends threw their arms toward me from where they slept on a low cot beside my hospital bed. So exhausted, these angel women, barely able to keep their heavy eyes open as they reached under my pajama top and swept their fingertips across my trembling back—at midnight, two in the morning, four thirty, and again at five. And that was on a good night.

Jill, my closest friend since the second grade, usually so perky and tireless in spite of a demanding job in advertising sales and two young kids, now bleary-eyed and slumped, hair gathered on her head in a pineapple-top ponytail. Lovely Jane, my go-to style guru who never seemed to mind my copycat attempts—*Tell me where you got those boots! What's the name of that lipstick?*—at once turned hospital drab in frayed sweatpants, her perfectly arched brows collapsed under worry weight. Lauren, the ever-meticulous mother of three and my stalwart escort to many of the surgeries, procedures, and scary medical tests that came along with my decades of heart transplant life, transformed by this California hospital stay into a cautious half-sleeping night owl in case she had to run and grab a nurse, flailing for her glasses at the faintest sound of my recurring whimper, "The pain . . . it's coming again . . ." Val, all steadiness and serenity even as my roommate during our grueling first year of law school, suddenly under extreme stress mixed with oncoming menopause—sweltering, self-spritzing frenetically with the spray bottle–fan combo she had brought with her all the way from Durham. And Ann, my hippie sister-in-law in platform flip-flops, her Mother Earth smile surrendering to tautened lips, wordless, just holding my hand.

Rougher than I had ever seen them, these five friends—along with four others—cared for me until the sun came up, showered quickly, if at all, and got right back to my bedside, cheerful and energetic. They pulled surprise gifts from their suitcases, anything to help me get through another day: buttery flannel pajamas with puppy-face print, peppermint lip gloss, lavender spray, a mud mask for two that transformed the hospital bed to a spa chaise one night. And then there were the rubber chickens and feather boas tacked to the wall, purple peace signs and Hawaiian leis hanging from the window shades—all purchased and arranged by Joy, my friend with a high-powered, executive-level job in Washington, DC, and yet also the one who flew to California to sleep beside me more nights than anyone else, always with a bag of new decorations to outdo the old, intent on transforming my room into its most ridiculous, death-distracting state.

But more than the tending and diverting, there was conversation—

our best talks yet. No filters. Last-chance candor. It was a time and place for unfastening. We got serious. Turned silly. Came clean. Worried. Mused. Raged. Laughed. Our honesty soared with purposeful abandon, answering a call of necessity that challenged each of us: *If not now, when?* We dove into truths and discoveries about ourselves, our husbands, our children, and our group of friends that lit the space around us to shimmering, no matter how alarming the signs that time was running out on my heart. Suspended in this desperately enchanted bubble, we found a new way to talk about life.

And when death did come up, in what were the frankest conversations of all, it was clear that no friend wanted me to die on her watch.

But neither did she want it to happen when she was not by my side.

Intense hours were spent together over the span of two and a half months—friend to friend, with unprecedented privacy for long stretches during the day and late into the night, and the sense that time was so short we absolutely could not delay going deep and learning from one another. Because, after all, every time one of these women left my California hospital room and flew home, she assumed she might never see me again.

This is the story of what that assumption brought out in each of us: our finest yet.

The result was transcendent.

1

Our words are winding down. There are silences, which means one of us is going to suggest we call it a night. And I'm thinking, *Okay, here it comes, it's got to come now*—a question from Joy that I should be prepared for, but I'm not.

She gets up from the couch and stands in front of me, puts her hands on her hips, and, yes, just as I thought: "How about if I sleep in your room tonight? It might make you feel more comfortable."

I look up at her and force a grin, closemouthed.

I'm buying time here. A quick answer could hurt her feelings.

Joy extends her arms, and I grab hold as she pulls me to my feet with a heave-ho. "Hey, look at that," she says, pointing, and I turn to see the deep well in the sofa cushion left by my arms-around-knees position.

"Guess I haven't moved in a while."

Joy nods. She and I both know that I didn't protest when she told me to *stay put* at lunchtime and fetched us each a yogurt from the fridge, and then again when dinner came and she carried into the family room two bowls of soup on a tray.

"So how 'bout it? Bunk up tonight?" she asks again, this time do-
ing the raised eyebrow thing that prompts me to put my hands on her
shoulders and say *I'm fine* and make a little joke about how, with Scott
away on a business trip, I want to take advantage of the rare occasion
when the remote control is mine, all mine.

It's a flimsy excuse, I know. But it's the best I can do on the spot.

Joy keeps on, "I hereby cede the remote control to you, my friend,
and may you watch *The Real Housewives of New York* until your brain
melts—won't bother me a bit. I've got a pile of work I planned on at-
tacking in bed tonight anyway."

At midnight? After a day like this?

I don't believe her.

But, then, she doesn't believe me either. I am not one to care a whit
about the remote, and I've never once seen the *Real Housewives* of any-
where. And Joy knows it.

"What if I put on *The Kardashians?*" I say, teasing her with the guilty
TV pleasure we've both fessed up to following with odd fascination.

"Then I'll hope it's a rerun."

"Oh, you watch those too—admit it," I say, trying to keep the ban-
ter going because it feels—for the moment, at least—like *us*. But each
successive comeback is an energy drain. We're both so weary, even our
kidding words drop to almost whispers.

And now we're moving through the family room and on toward the
kitchen—fluffing one cushion and not another, grabbing two mugs
and leaving two glasses, turning off random lights. We float, wide-
eyed, absent, leaving imperfection in our wake.

Without saying out loud to each other in agreement, *Let's leave the
rest 'til morning*, we drift to the base of the staircase as one. Here, we
find Joy's overnight bag at our feet, unmoved from the spot where she
dropped it in deliberate haste after coming straight from the airport.
"And don't ask me if I want to head to the guest room to freshen up,"
she instructed early this morning after a quick hello hug on arrival at
my front door, the *New York Times* from the driveway tucked under her

arm, "because I don't. Just tell me which couch to sit on and let's get to it." I cocked my head to the side and smiled, not knowing quite what to make of this whirl of bossiness that was now spinning itself out of its winter coat and heading toward the kitchen, calling out, "Let's make tea!"

This was my friend Joy—exaggerated.

I'd noticed the same a week earlier when I called her at the office and interrupted her pressure cooker workday with an awkward ask: "Here's the thing—on the sixth, Scott has to go away for three days, ah . . . do you think maybe you could . . ."

"Done!" She didn't even pause to check her calendar.

"But, Joy, wait . . . let me just tell you, it's not going to be any fun. I'm at my worst and—"

"I'm *there*. End of discussion. Email me the exact dates. And now I . . . I'm sorry, but I have to, uh . . ."

"You're in a meeting."

"Sort of, I mean, it's okay, I can talk now if . . ."

"Go, go! I'm good—really!"

And so began the dance—the gliding around each other, watchful, careful.

Uncharacteristically choreographed. I wasn't *good* at all, and Joy's executive-level job was not flexible enough to allow her to just drop out of the office on a week's notice.

We were not ourselves with each other. But how could we be? My transplanted heart was coming to its abrupt end. It was not a case of *Let's try this medicine* or *Let's watch and wait*. No—it was over. There was no definitive bright spot of hope, only retransplant—*if* my heart had enough beats left to get me there.

And *if* I chose to let it try.

This was the subject matter we would take on for three uninterrupted days together: whether I would choose to rise up one last time and brave the harrowing ordeal and risks of a retransplant. It was so far beyond anything we had combed through or sorted out in the past, even considering how adept Joy had become at digging into the nitty-gritty of medical crises in her role as good friend to a heart transplant patient for more than two decades. It would require of each of us a new kind of poise—an affected one—and a backbone so straight and sturdy it could support a basis for communication we'd never had use for in the past: sparing each other.

With her high-energy, can-do determination to be the best friend ever—at my side 24/7, taking Scott's place by listening, reasoning, and weighing the terrible options with me—Joy strove to keep hidden the deep worry and sadness that had her dabbing her eyes right until the cab dropped her at the bottom of my driveway. By the time she rang my doorbell, the wad of tissues peeking out from her fist and the red-ringed eyes that greeted mine were the only outward sign of her concern, masked by her otherwise bright smile and enthusiastic embrace.

And me, with my *I'm fine* nonsense, greeting Joy in a way that would put her at ease—dressed in exercise leggings and a bright-colored running top, as if I might head to the gym at any moment. I even broke my weeklong stint of bedroom-slipper shuffling with a purposeful lacing-up of well-worn Nikes, the ones I ran miles in until about a month ago when intense pain started shooting down my arms at random moments and my doctor told me, "Maybe you should lay off exercise until we know what's going on."

I hadn't had reason to put on my running sneakers again until today, for Joy.

For the performance I would do for her, the high kicks, twirls, and dips to show how fine I was.

There I was this morning at the front door, with my freshly washed, bouncy hair, a little mascara and blush, and a lip-gloss smile that I stretched wider than usual. This way, I hoped, I might create more room in my airway to better handle the breathlessness that accompanied even the smallest expenditure of energy. Like when I followed Joy's quickstep dash into the kitchen, trailing behind in slow motion, hoping she wouldn't notice the lag. By the time I joined her, she'd already flipped the lid off the teakettle and had turned to the sink to fill it. I grabbed hold of the nearest countertop for support. She swung back around and I let go in a flash.

"I have to say, you look great . . . mmm, maybe a little on the thin side, though," she said, placing the kettle down and turning her head this way and that, taking me in with a long look.

"I've been eating fine."

I haven't been.

Joy's cell phone rang just then. She ran back to the staircase to retrieve it from her bag and called out, "I gotta pick this up, it's the office. But it should be quiet after this—no more calls for the rest of the day."

Joy had a team of nearly seven hundred people working under her at Fannie Mae. Her decade-long senior vice president role in the Washington, DC, office had shifted with the fallout of the housing crisis, and she now found herself at the very center of the national programs to restructure mortgages and help people stay in their homes. She rose tirelessly to the challenge of round-the-clock hours and daunting demands, often sitting in hot seats in front of US Treasury big shots who would make a less stalwart VP melt. Always quick to use a baseball reference, Joy would tell me that she strove to "knock it out of the park" when it came to her work, and this meant overpreparing and overperfecting to achieve an outcome that reverberated beyond corporate walls.

Her work mattered on a grand scale, certainly, and also a personal one. Joy told me many times how deeply connected she felt to the results of her efforts—to the thousands and thousands of people who could benefit from or be hurt by the policies she helped inform and shape. After all, she herself grew up in a barely middle-class family that lived on an income that might easily have placed them in the same financial perils she now sought to relieve for others.

So when she picked up her cell phone early this morning—and then again at eleven, twice in the late afternoon, and one more time after dinner—"Oops, it's the Treasury again, I'll take this in the other room"—I was not at all surprised. Part of what I love and admire about

Joy is exactly this: her unstoppable devotion, both as a working person and as a friend. She's one of those rare women who somehow manages to succeed in filling these two roles to fullest capacity without showing a hint of strain. Friends, as well as the tall stacks of work on Joy's desk, get the absolute best out of her. But this comes at a personal cost, of course.

"I'm a giver, what can I say?" is how she has responded to my frequent urging to ease up on her work schedule after consecutive weeks of punishing business travel, or at least to say no to those out-of-town friends of friends who ask last minute to stay at her apartment for a few days of sightseeing in Washington the weekend she finally returns home. (She welcomes them instead.)

And now I see in front of me again a worn-out but ever-willing Joy. This time, though, *I* am the one taking her giving, having stolen from her one full workday so far and, at this late hour, some much-needed sleep time as well.

I reach for her overnight bag at the bottom of the staircase and am met with a grab for the handle and a squawk along the lines of *Are you kidding me?*

"You're my guest," I say. "And . . . your bad shoulder."

"Uh, excuse me, Miss Manners. May I point out . . . your *heart*?"

"I can climb the stairs in my own house, Joy. I do it two, three times a day carrying all kinds of things—dental floss, a roll of toilet paper, the occasional elephant," I cluck, in a small effort at poking fun, but at once I feel the weight of the lie. I *can* climb, yes, but increasingly it requires a mix of concentration and courage to handle the sputtering heart that awaits me at the top.

I gesture for her to go first—"After you, my dear!"—trying to sound nonchalant, but hoping with all hope that she will go slowly.

And she does.

Very slowly.

Stepping up and then up again, I notice Joy's ankles peeking out from the bottom of her chinos and see that they're quite swollen. The bone that normally protrudes from the outside of each ankle is submerged by waterlog. Joy has complained to me lately about puffiness that hangs on after air travel—but this morning's flight was only an hour long.

Significant water retention in the extremities is a sign of heart failure.

This is where my mind goes—automatically. I can't help but think medically.

Of course, I've been evaluating my own ankles before bed each night. Pressing along the bone and then up a few inches toward my calf, I'm horrified by the deep imprints my fingers leave behind—like pokes into soft clay at first, then refilling slowly with the overload of body fluid that I know signals big trouble.

"If you push your finger into the base of your ankle, does it leave an indentation for a few seconds?" I asked Joy a few weeks ago when she told me that she couldn't fit her feet back into her loafers after a flight to Detroit.

"I don't know."

"Well, try it and see."

"Nah, never mind. It's just my Italian-grandma genes. A pinch of salt and a few hours in a plane, and I balloon up five pounds."

How easy it was for her to dismiss my concern. It didn't matter that I had long been Joy's first call when symptoms like postnasal drip with severe headache showed up. "Is this a sinus infection, Dr. Amy?" she'd ask, and I would dispense advice along with my recommendation for a specific antibiotic, citing swiftly from memory the generic and brand names, milligram dosage, duration of treatment, and side effects. "Tell your doctor you need *this*," I would say. I could hear Joy actually applauding through the phone; she marveled at the depth of my medical knowledge, and she enjoyed the benefits of my advice whenever she felt something brewing.

But when it came to puffy extremities, my knowledge and vigilance did not apply to Joy. She was healthy. Normal. She and I could never look at puffy ankles the same way.

Reaching the top step now, Joy's legs move out of sight—and mind.

A racing heartbeat takes me over, as I knew it would. It's a relief to see her make an unhurried left turn and amble down the hall at a lazy pace; I may just be able to catch up.

She puts down her bag and exhales, "Long day," and shoots me a sly smile, shifting her eyes repeatedly toward my bedroom door as I approach—a signal to me that she's still up for sleeping in my room.

"Something going on with your eyes there, Joy?" I imitate her with exaggerated side-glances.

"Whatever do you mean? I'm just giving the ol' eyeballs some exercise . . . and my bushy eyebrows too!" she jokes, wiggling her face like Groucho Marx. But within seconds our smiles falter.

It's time to go to bed.

Joy's last crusade has to be here and now, or not at all.

She decelerates. Pauses. Blinks twice and opens her mouth a few seconds before anything comes out. "Seriously, my friend—you don't have to be alone."

"Oh—but I do."

She folds her arms and sighs. "Why? You don't need to prove anything. I know how strong you are. Take a break from it tonight, just this once. I'm here. Let me help make this a nice, easy night for you."

A nice, easy night?

"Joy—I'm *sick*!"

My words hang in the air.

She drops her head. "I know," she whispers.

But she doesn't.

Not really.

What Joy knows is the medical reality revealed three weeks ago by an invasive cardiac exam: that unless I get a second heart transplant soon, I'm going to die. But in all the hours we spent today in deep conversation, I did not tell her anything about how this dying feels.

I lift my gaze to the far end of the hallway and stare drearily as if into dense fog. "Look, Joy. I'm . . . It's . . . it's like my grandmother.

She was old, had a really sick heart. Wore one of those emergency-call necklaces. She pressed the button on it one day and the paramedics got there pretty fast, but they couldn't save her. They said it was one heart attack too many. And everyone at the funeral was all, *Oh, she's dead, oh, we've lost her.* Death, death, death, you know? As if that's what happened to her."

I lean against the wall and slump. I've been standing too long.

Joy steps toward me. "You okay?"

I hold up my hand: *Stop.*

"But death—that wasn't what happened, really. What happened to my grandmother was the damn heart attack that made her press that button—crushing pain in the chest must've taken the breath right out of her, collapsed her to the floor, poor thing, terrified. I heard they found her in a pool of diarrhea and vomit. *That's* what my grandma felt at the end. *That's* what happened to her. Death is just the thing that happens to the people you leave behind."

I move away from the wall and will myself to stand straight.

"I'm grandma on the floor, Joy. You sleeping in my room is not going to make my night any easier."

Her eyes fill instantly. A tear escapes, and she turns her head to hide it beneath the curve of her blond bob.

The grief has become too heavy, too real—for both of us. Our dance of sparing each other isn't going to work anymore, so we stop. And all I can think to do in this moment at the catty-corner of bedroom and guest room is to say, "I love you, and I can't tell you how much I appreciate . . ."

Up shoots her hand, sweeping toward my nose, away, away, which I understand to mean *Shut. Up. With. That.*

So I do.

Wiping our eyes, we smile at each other—this time for real. Two bedroom doors close simultaneously, our faces disappearing behind them.

Click.

I am alone.

And now I have to try to not die tonight.

THIS ALL STARTED about two months ago, with what I thought was a worn-out pillow. I lay down in bed one night and sensed that my body was on a downward slope with my head positioned lower than my feet, causing my insides to bunch up around my chest and throat. It was hard to breathe.

I told Scott it was time we both got new pillows.

But the same thing continued to happen night after night, no matter the feather count beneath my head. Breathing my way into sleep became fraught.

"It feels like the room is tilted," I told Scott, jumping from our bed and squatting beside it to see if the plane was level. "Maybe the floor is settling on a slant or something."

He shrugged—"Seems fine to me"—and curled into sleep position.

After all, I didn't say anything about feeling out of breath.

I grabbed my pillow and tossed it by the footboard at the other end of the bed. I lay down, this time in reverse position, predicting that my head would feel higher than my feet this way. But within seconds I was up again—I shot up, actually—to a fully upright sitting position.

I was gasping.

After a minute or two, I caught my breath and struggled quickly to settle my mind before extreme worry set in. I was not going to let myself get really scared—not yet. I did a brief body check: My heart wasn't pounding. I was not sweating or in pain. I was able to breathe in this small moment, sitting up.

Calm, Amy, calm.

I knew well that no good could come from getting a transplanted heart all worked up.

I willed myself to refocus.

Maybe if I open my mouth really wide there will be a better flow of air, I told myself, holding down the creeping panic. I snapped open my jaw to its widest stretch.

Nope.

I thought about propping a bolster pillow behind my back so I could sleep sitting up, but that would be giving in, damn it. I was going to lie down and breathe, because not being able to do so would bring to mind the frightening possibility that my transplanted heart was starting to fail—and the vivid memory that fueled this thought. Breathlessness in bed had also been the first symptom I had felt twenty-six years earlier when I was a busy law student who dismissed the nightly wheezing and gurgling in my chest as some kind of allergy. But I had been wrong: my symptoms back then were actually due to my heart's diminished pumping capacity and its fearsome consequence—fluid in my lungs.

In bed with Scott all these years later, I cringed as I contemplated whether to force myself to be more accurate in my body assessment this time around. I was fifty years old now, not twenty-five, and after nearly three decades of living and absorbing the teachings of transplant cardiology, it would require more effort to self-deceive than to be honest.

I knew too much.

Am I dying again? I could not stop the question from crossing my mind, but rather than answer, I heaved it aside and vowed not to give in to this breathing thing.

And even when additional ominous symptoms popped up over the next few days and weeks, I remained determined to rise above what was shaping up to be a troubling combination. To give in was unthinkably scary.

"You're not out of breath—*are you?*" my doctor asked when I finally called to report that I felt palpitations during and after my morning workouts. His question sent a chill through me—because I knew at once the deadly diagnosis it prodded: heart failure. I worried that I would be letting us both down if I said yes.

"No."

He sent me for some cardiac tests anyway. And after the first round,

which showed marked arrhythmia, we weren't much closer to a defin-
itive diagnosis.

"Maybe this is just how old transplanted hearts behave," was the
best he could offer me by way of interpretation. Sure, I reasoned, trans-
planted hearts are prone to skips and runs of fast beats; it was logical
that these aberrations might occur increasingly over time. But there
was no way to know with certainty what was happening to mine with-
out further invasive testing, since there was hardly any data to compare
me with other patients at three decades post–heart transplant. There
were not enough of us alive this long after surgery to create a useful
cohort. I was an outlier, my doctor confirmed.

It was anyone's guess why I had survived so far beyond the ten-year
if you are really lucky life expectancy given to me by doctors when my
natural-born twenty-five-year-old heart suddenly become so sick it had
to be severed from my chest and replaced.

The one time I pressed my doctor to explain my longevity, even he
hesitated awkwardly, scrambling to come up with something: "Uh,
good clean living?"

But I had known lots of clean-living transplant recipients who
fought for survival with the same devotion to their donor hearts as I
did, and they'd all died.

I feel the weight of this again tonight as I stand beside my empty
bed alone and face the breathlessness to come: the transplant years that
have made me a mysterious outlier have also made me a vanishing
one. In the month leading up to Joy's visit, my symptoms progressed
with dangerous speed from nightly breathing trouble to ominous pal-
pitations and, most recently, to a sharp, radiating pain through my
arms and shoulders. And additional testing in the wake of my doctor's
old-transplanted-heart speculation confirmed my worst fears: that my
heart is riddled with vasculopathy—a dreaded, incurable transplant ar-
tery disease.

The condition is precarious, which means that anything can hap-
pen at any time. *But please, don't let it happen tonight*—not with Scott

away and Joy sleeping in the next room. If my heart suddenly gave out, it would devastate Joy irremediably and Scott would never forgive himself for leaving.

It would be no one's fault, of course. It would just be bad timing that landed Scott at an important out-of-town meeting that he couldn't avoid. He is one partner of three in a small candy business he started up recently with two former colleagues. The very foundations of the company—sourcing, production, and distribution—will be worked out over these few days away. He absolutely has to be there.

And Joy—brave Joy, coming here in his absence!—is an enormous relief to Scott. They'd met in law school at the University of Pennsylvania and were great friends long before she and I became close. When I visited Scott on weekends, I was cautious of this wonderful Joy he talked about so animatedly—the girl who, he'd told me in admiring detail, had just created and orchestrated three hours of Wedding Olympics at a nearby park for a friend who was getting married and was worried that her out-of-town guests would have a ho-hum day before the evening party. The range of Joy's invented competitions included the Toilet Seat Dash (for which the amazing Joy brought in two toddler-size potties as props), with "husband" running some twenty yards to lift the seat up and then "wife" following suit, making her dash to put it down, and so on.

"I can't wait for you to really get to know her," Scott said.

I could.

It was no wonder my first imaginings of Joy came with a mixture of wariness and jealousy. This creative, energetic, outgoing gal-pal looked to me like perpetual competition, especially since I was hours away at NYU law school while she was impressing my boyfriend with her high-spirited amiability all week long—in that *friend* kind of way, of course.

Looking at Joy today, though—sitting on the couch with me at absolute attention, leaning in toward my every word with an expression of complete earnestness and caring—I felt the urge to snap my eyes closed and shake my head like an Etch A Sketch to clear away the thought that my now close friend would have been the type to move in on Scott between my visits to Penn. But Joy and I were in our early twenties back when we first met; having a few drinks too many and winding up with someone else's boyfriend for a night was not an unusual happening. No one was married; the consequence of dalliance was simply drama, not divorce. And love was just— What *was* love, anyway?

This is what Scott would show me by astounding example.

We'd been dating less than one year when I was rushed by ambulance to what was then Columbia Presbyterian Hospital (now NewYork-Presbyterian/Columbia University Medical Center) in New York, where I was told that I was dying fast and needed a heart transplant. It was 1988 and Scott was twenty-six, one year older than I. He knelt on the floor beside my ICU bed and asked me to marry him, diamond ring in hand, even though a defibrillator cart careened into my room with terrifying regularity, just barely in time to shock my heart from deathly rhythms. By courageous proposal, this shining, perfectly healthy young man was committing himself to a woman who doctors had predicted might live only ten years after transplant, optimistically speaking—if she even survived to receive a matching donor heart. And yet Scott insisted on marrying me, fully willing to become a widower by the time he turned thirty-six.

What kind of a twenty-six-year-old guy does that?

"I'm lovable, but not *that* lovable" has been the line I've routinely added as a jaunty kick when unfolding the drama of my engagement story for someone new. It always gets the chuckle I intend, but I mean it in all seriousness: How could I be worth this kind of sacrifice?

"Scott's love for you is not like normal average love, you know that, don't you?" Joy said this afternoon, lifting her pen from a writing pad and looking up at me. We'd been making a list of the pros and cons of going for a retransplant—or not.

"Yes. I think about it all the time."

She put the pad on the coffee table in front of us and folded her hands. "Okay, so how does this figure into your choice?"

"I guess you're thinking that if I say no to a second transplant, I'm essentially saying to Scott, *I choose death over the chance to have more years with you.*"

"He might see it that way, yeah."

But I knew this wasn't so.

The last couple of weeks had forced Scott and me to have some of our most difficult talks, not that our discussions over the years had been easy; my state of constant illness since my transplant had us talking about life and death in ways most couples would never have to. "Am I going to take this one on?" was not a question arising now for the first time in the face of retransplant. The piling up of hospitalizations, emergency room visits, and ambulance rides over the nearly twenty-six transplant years had made each battle call into an option to be discussed rather than an automatic mission on my part. And although, for Scott, anything that saved my life was always worth doing, he understood how, for me, there needed to be a conscious choice because the battle was in *my* body—and so was the suffering.

I picked up the writing pad and glanced at the bullet points Joy had jotted down. "Look at these cons. Scott has lived every one of them right along with me. He wants me to do the transplant anyway, of course; he wants me with him. But he says he can see why I might say no."

The list set it out clearly: this second transplant would be far from a cure-all. At best, it promises to be a continuation of what has been a miraculously long and gratefully lived—but terribly sick—heart transplant life. Scott knows that I would have a much shorter life expectancy this time around and that the increased levels of immunosuppressive transplant medicines would bring on an even greater number of serious illnesses. My quality of life would be more trying than it already was. So, while Scott told me with tear-filled eyes that he hoped I would forge on with retransplant, he acknowledged that this was asking a lot of me. But I didn't think so—not with regard to him, anyway. Scott had every right to ask me for the moon.

"When he proposed in that hospital room twenty-five years ago, it was incredible—I mean, that love could be this deep and true! But Joy—and let's keep this just between us, okay?—it's also something I've had to measure myself against. I double-check myself for selfishness all the time, even with small things, like, *Oh, I should pick up the dirty clothes Scott left by his side of the bed because, after all, he married me even with a heart transplant.*"

She laughed.

"No, I mean it. And sometimes I get really tough on myself and ask, *Okay, if roles were reversed and it had been young Scott in a hospital bed with a short and very sick life ahead, would I have married him?*"

"You would, right?"

"Of course, yes. But I'm answering this question *now*, as a grown woman. I never thought about it even once when I twenty-five. See? Selfish."

I felt the familiar pang: *I can never be as good a person as Scott.*

Comparing myself to him always leaves me feeling the imbalance in what we've done for each other. I haven't had (and probably will never have) the opportunity to commit for Scott an act so great, so all encompassing and lifelong, as his marriage proposal. Lately, though, I've been thinking that if I say yes to the transplant, maybe it could be *my* big sacrifice for love, like he made years ago. But then, every one of our conversations over the last few days has ended with Scott insisting that he absolutely does not want me to take on a second transplant for his sake—and I believe him.

"You've got to let all of that go," Joy said, meeting my eyes. "Scott is maybe the most thoughtful and giving person I know. Who can hold themselves up against that? You're plenty good, Amy. Plenty. Everything you do every day shows that you adore him."

Yeah. But when he left on his business trip this morning, I didn't catch his arm, pull him close, and say, *Scotty, I'm going to do it.*

I SLIDE UNDER the sheets and launch into the only thing that can carry me through these breathless nights: distraction—by the diligent, even obsessive, and sometimes kooky processes that I sometimes think of as applied magic. I am not proud of this. It is not in my nature to turn to nonsense ritual. But when you're given ten unlikely years of transplant heartbeats, along with lifelong nonnegotiable medications that can and eventually will invite dangerous infections and cancers to take hold within you repeatedly, optimism just doesn't cut it.

When the fates of life shine a spotlight sharp and terrible on something that can't ever be fixed, you might just put on a pair of sunglasses. Not because the muted tones will make things look like they're not so bad after all, as that's impossible; you've glimpsed the hard, vivid truth, and it stays with you like the blot that endures after looking wide-eyed into a solar eclipse. No, you slide behind those large, dark lenses and become, at key moments, someone unrecognizable—even to yourself.

The direst circumstances rarely connect you with your deepest essence; rather, they distance you from it. And this makes it easier to go on.

What does a woman do when she's lying on the procedure table, about to have her seventy-fifth heart biopsy—an invasive cardiac transplant exam that becomes exponentially more complex and dangerous over time? There she is, fully awake while a doctor snips off pieces of her heart muscle by inserting a catheter with a razor-tip pincer end through her neck vein and into her left ventricle—in and out, in and out, snip-snip-snip, again and again.

How does she get herself through?

She recites poetry, that's how. From memory.

Sometimes silently, sometimes aloud.

And she doesn't give a crap who hears. She's just getting by.

When my heart jumps as the biopsy catheter lands midventricle, I close my eyes and start: "Invictus." *Out of the night that covers me, black as the pit from pole to pole, I thank whatever gods may be for my unconquerable* . . .

Pluck!

The doctor tears one piece of heart tissue, then retracts the catheter from the center of my heart and pulls it out through my neck. He deposits the sample in a sterile container for later examination under a microscope that will reveal either normal cells or aberrant ones that indicate rejection of the donor heart—a disease process that can be treatable, or unstoppable and ultimately fatal.

"We got one," the doctor chirps, and stuffs the line back in for another go. He will have to extract four sizeable pieces to complete the full procedure, and not every pluck is a successful one. Sometimes it takes him eighteen tries to get good-quality tissue samples.

One time, it required two full recitations of all six pages of T. S. Eliot's "The Love Song of J. Alfred Prufrock" to hold on during a biopsy that took twenty-two heart plucks to complete.

And Scott had thought I was memorizing all of those stanzas— mumbling tricky sentences to myself in the kitchen while the pasta boiled—for no good reason.

I do not share my mind routines with Scott, or with anyone. Given my age and transplant years, I feel people expect me to be better. More stalwart. Less kooky. I should be well poised in my role of fantastic survivor; it's all got to be second nature to me by now, right? And because I continue to beat the odds so seamlessly, I stand as an example who gives others hope that many years from now, when they grow old and, inevitably, get hit with some insurmountable health challenge, perhaps they too can lie on exam tables with grace and stretch their expiration date by two decades.

"Whenever I've got a huge challenge at work and I just can't rally myself, I think of you," Joy said to me today, "and I get perspective and strength. I'm constantly in awe of you—how you tackle whatever tries to knock you down, you're my—"

"Inspiration? Oh please, please don't call me that," I said, hunching forward as if she had suddenly placed a load on my back.

In bed now, my mind returns to this conversation and I round it out with the truth: *If you knew what I am about to do now that you are out of sight, Joy, you might come up with different words for me, like* terrified *and* desperate.

This is the Amy no one knows.

And now I must collapse into ritual—not because I'm prone to compulsive behaviors, but rather because some things are just too horrifying, like the need for a second heart transplant.

Tonight, Joy, I count windowpanes.

Lying on my right side, I see four of them in direct view: glass separated by white wooden dividers. I will fill these four spaces with air.

Let's see: Four is my favorite number. Sixteen is even better since it is four squared, so I will breathe in and out four times on each pane, moving my gaze clockwise as I go from one to the next.

I want to believe that this will bring sufficient oxygen into my body, but as skilled as I am at narrowing my thoughts to focus only on windowpanes or lines of beautiful verse, I have never been successful at subjecting my mind to delusion; I know for sure that even my most concentrated attention cannot work real magic here. I am just trying to get by.

I begin.

Upper left corner: breathe in deep, hold, and out. I repeat this four times, telling myself that it does not matter that my heart is sick and cannot pump anywhere near normal capacity anymore; if I concentrate hard enough, air will flow through me.

And again, with stronger intent: upper right pane this time. Breathe in, hold, and out. In and out.

This is not working. I need more air.

I move my eyes quickly to the lower right square—in-out-in-out . . .
I can't breathe, I can't breathe, I can't breathe.
I heave my body up to sitting and start to cry.
I give in! Gasp. *I give up!*
I am not brave enough to watch myself die this way.
This is not a choice.
I have to live.
I have to try for this retransplant.
But, oh my God, I just can't—
I can't . . .
I know too well what is ahead of me if I move forward with this choice.

I am weeping now as I grab the bolster from Scott's side of the bed to prop it behind my back. I will sleep sitting up.

And with tomorrow's earliest sun, I will look through the window-panes that failed me and hope to find my first name spelled out in the angles of bare tree branches set against the gray February sky. So many mornings for so many years, my eyes found their way to a distinct *A*, an *M*, and, less easily, a *Y*. And when they did, it felt like the jutting branches were holding me up with the power of their centennials, keeping my body from plunging into the depths where old transplanted hearts are fated to go.

But just this morning, I thought I saw the angles connect in new formation as I listened to the rumble roll of Scott's suitcase fade in the hallway. They said to me, *Sorry, Amy, we tried.*

THREE YEARS EARLIER

Freshman move-in day at Oberlin College was drawing to a close.
Orientation activities for parents had ended, and Scott and I were walking Casey back to his dorm.

Then, suddenly, a whoosh.

A jolt of dizziness.

My heart hammered erratically in my chest, my throat—BANG-BANG . . . BANGBANG . . . BANG—but I kept walking.

I didn't want Casey to see.

We reached the dorm lobby, and I whispered to Scott as he held the door for me, "My heart's not right. I'll tell you in the car."

Then there were three flights to climb to Casey's room.

Oh please, oh please, let me make it there.

I didn't know to what or whom I was pleading.

Halfway up, I had to wipe my forehead; I shouldn't be sweating like this.

"I love you, my Caseyboy," I heard myself say once we reached the third floor lounge and I hugged him close. "I'm so proud of you."

Scott went in for his hug—and we were off.

To the nearest hospital.

I called my transplant doctor in New York on the way, and he said there was a good hospital in Cleveland, and yes, I should go there immediately. He didn't doubt me when I told him, "This is not a case of college-drop-off-day emotion."

"You're no hypochondriac," he said. "Go to the ER."

Once Scott and I had driven beyond the mob of parents and kids saying their good-byes, I could let the tears come, finally. "Whatever this is, it's bad . . ."

And I was right.

Something changed in my heartbeat that day, and it terrified me—though not because I saw it as the clear harbinger of my heart's demise; I wouldn't come to realize this until years later, when I was able to look back and put together the pieces that would show themselves cryptically, little symptom by little symptom, from that day forward.

No, the fright of this moment on college move-in day was due to the eerie actualization of an imagining I'd been pushing from my mind while packing up Casey's bedroom: that my heart might sense his departure for college and, noting the elapsed urgency of keeping a mommy alive for her no-longer-young son, wind down from super-survival mode.

Crazy? What was crazy was that I was alive to see Casey enter college.

I had only five years of predicted life expectancy left when Scott and I adopted him as an infant. But there hadn't been any trace of deathly transplant disease in my donor heart at that time, and my doctor seemed to indicate that I'd moved past the most dangerous early post-transplant period, saying things like "Who told you only ten years?" (he did) and "You could very well be one of the lucky ones who lives two decades or more." So, Scott and I went into parenthood with sober optimism; perhaps I could live to raise our boy for many years, but in any case Scott would play an exceptionally active role as a father and would take over with confidence as a single parent if need be.

It was a fate beyond all reasonable hope to find myself picking through my eighteen-year-old son's closet, calling out, "Hey, Case, do you want to take your winter boots now or pick them up at Thanksgiving?" It had always frightened me how much I adored him; I was never able to settle casually into the day-to-day rhythm of mother and son because our time together was too fragile. And now here I was with my boy turned bearded young man. How was it that I hadn't died when he was in kindergarten?

One explanation: my heart eked out an extraordinary feat of endurance because year after year there was a boy who called me Mommy.

But Mommy had turned to Mom.

And I was packing my nearly two decades of motherhood into cardboard boxes carefully and deliberately—warm quilt (check), shower flip-flops (check), Band-Aids (check).

Even without actually laying eyes upon what Casey and I were doing in his room that day, anyone—or any heart—listening in on our words and to the squeaky sound of package tape stretching over box tops would know what was happening: A young man was leaving home. And his mother was helping.

"I hope my heart didn't hear," I said to a few friends when all the boxes were stacked up and ready to go.

I was only half kidding.

"Hearts can't hear, right?"

Right, they assured me.

And we laughed.

But, just a few days later, preliminary cardiac tests in Cleveland (followed by many more in New York) showed that my heart function had declined—all of a sudden. Significantly.

And it would continue to worsen in small but sure increments over the weeks and months to come. As time passed, the how, why, and when of disease progression became muddled and complicated. Compounded and confused.

But I would never forget where the end of my heart began: with Casey leaving for college.

Coincidence?

Maybe if I'd wound up in an emergency room a few months after his departure, I could have chalked it up to chance.

Even a few weeks' lag time would have given me cause for doubt.

But to have my heart show its first sign of failure on college move-in day? On the exact day I parted with the son I'd raised to near independence?

I'm not saying hearts have ears, but . . .

Well, maybe I am.

2

_____

The phone rings and Jill's name pops up on the caller ID. I'm thinking of ignoring it. Joy left my house only an hour ago, after all, and I've barely begun to wind down from our weekend of nonstop conversation. But if I don't pick up, Jill will try my cell phone— and if that fails, she'll call Scott at the office to let him know I've gone MIA—and then he will call me at once (I'll answer this time) and ex- hale a plea in a somber tone, "Don't do that to your friends."

I reach for the receiver. "Hey," I say, infusing as little sound as possible.

"Ames? Ames?" Jill can't hear me. She's on a morning dash from Grand Central Terminal to her office in Rockefeller Center. There are sirens in the background. Truck horns. The sound of heavy rain. "You there?"

"Here," I say, a little louder this time.

"Okay, good. I know Scott's still away, so . . . I'm comin' over tomor- row morning, all right?"

"Mmmm—no. Sorry. I just . . . I'd rather be by myself. Thanks, though."

"Aw, lemme come. We'll just hang, no presh, okay?"

"Jill, I really—"

"*I'm not hearing you!*" she says, slipping into falsetto. "*Tra-la-la-la-la . . .*"

"I really would prefer if you didn't."

"No, no, no, no, no. Just want to see you. No big deal. I'll be over around nine."

I shake my head—no way I'm going to win this one. I tell her let's make it nine thirty, and she shouts, "Yay!"

"I'M JUST A body," Jill announces, moving past me in sneakers, *squeak-squeaking* across the wooden floor before plopping down onto my living room couch. "I brought some work with me and I'm going to sit here for a few hours. You don't have to talk to me. You don't even have to *look* at me—I know I'm a mess, sorry . . ." Her dark hair is damp around the temples and pulled back into a high ponytail. "I just did the elliptical. Hope I don't—I don't smell, do I?" she says, sniffing under each arm.

I settle into a chair a few feet away. "Can't tell from here."

"Well, you just stay where you are, 'cause I'm a-stinkin' all right," she chirps in that put-on voice of hers—or, really, ours. Jill is my oldest and dearest friend. We've been close since the second grade, and the years have allowed us a language of our own or, more specifically, playful sarcasm with a goofy cadence. Even picking up the phone gets us right to it: "Je-je-*Jell-O!*" is how we usually answer each other's calls. There is rarely an exchange that doesn't turn us into cornballs—trading familiar gag lines that never wear thin, the silliest nonsense that brings us back to the giggles of Mrs. West's elementary school class, where we shared a cubby for our gym sneakers and cheated at hopscotch on the blacktop at recess.

Jill now works in advertising sales and is a crackerjack—highly accomplished, seasoned, and respected. But even when we were girls, she had a way about her. Our seventh grade drama teacher summed up

Jill's essence perfectly, announcing to the class after an hour of mostly clumsy scene reading: "Jill's got it."

I wasn't sure what she meant at the time, although I do remember agreeing with her, if silently: the friend I loved best was something special. It wasn't until some years after college that I came to understand that among Jill's greatest and most useful gifts were irresistibility and a knack for persuasiveness—tremendous assets that have distinguished her not only in advertising sales, but also in her suburban life as mother, wife, and well-liked gal in the community where we both live.

Jill is the only friend I know who has her own Cablevision repairman—got him to write down his personal cell phone number and email. One simple service call at her house and the guy was hers—no more interactions with the darn automated customer service. Jill's aplomb in slipping him twenty or thirty bucks was impressive, sure, but her real finesse was in translating that moment into years and years of on-call service. In big-brown-eyed, sweet-smiling form, my friend Jill could put her charm and smarts to work in any scenario.

And these are the graces she's brought with her into my living room this morning, just days after hearing the bad news about my transplanted heart. Jill is going to try to get me to do something; I know it.

Maybe it's just to talk things out? Nah. There's got to be more . . .

I watch for a sign of motive as she reaches into her tote bag and pulls out a few folders and then a laptop—calm, matter-of-fact. But her silence gives her away; ordinarily, Jill would be chatting me up about anything and everything, even if I didn't respond. "Want some distraction?" she has asked me many times in a multitude of tense medical moments, like in the waiting room before a heart biopsy or while speeding me to the hospital when I spiked a fever and Scott was out of town. She always comes up with something amusing to lure my attention away from whatever looms horrible and scary.

But not today. Jill is quiet, and this means she's concentrating.

We long ago admitted to each other that we're terrible multitaskers and need perfect silence when executing an important task. And here we are now, on the verge of something we've never approached before. The reality of my need for a retransplant looms, and each of us is hushed, focused inward. No doubt, Jill is poised for action.

I pull away from her in anticipation, slinking down in my chair with glazed, indifferent eyes while she opens a folder and pretends to concentrate on some papers there. And just then a memory comes to me—a detailed recollection from our treasure of shared experiences. I let my mind drift . . .

There we are, Jill and I, on a Saturday morning. We've met up at the blacktop we played on as kids. This time, though, we're junior high big shots, with one cigarette and a book of matches between us; it's our plan to try smoking for the first time, together.

"You light it."

"No, you light it."

"No. You!"

"You!"

Neither one of us can bring ourselves to strike a match. Jill has justification: sparks from a faulty fondue pot splattered on her when she was a toddler. But I'm just a big chicken when it comes to fire.

"I've got a for-real reason why I'm afraid," she tells me, pointing to a couple of tiny white spots on the side of her cheek. "You have to light it because I can't."

"But . . ."

"There's nothing stopping you from lighting one tiny little match. It's all in your head."

Jill was thirteen and methodical.

She stood with her fist pressed against her hip and looked down at the blacktop as if it were the saddest surface she'd ever seen—and I gave in.

I remember tearing out a single stem, closing the matchbook, and setting to it. But I slid the red tip reticently across the strike pad over and over again, until it slipped from my grasp and landed facedown in a puddle.

We howled with laughter, and the pressure evaporated. There we were, trying to be naughty. Cool. Rule-breaking. Smokin' in the schoolyard. But, really, we were just a couple of good girls from a safe little town on Long Island. We decided there and then: *This counts as trying smoking, okay?* Agreed.

We left the paraphernalia on the blacktop and walked home. No harm done.

I would always remember the day Jill got me to try to light a match; I wouldn't have done it for anyone else—but then, Jill had a way. And now here she is in my living room some thirty-five years later, telling me she's got an idea.

"So I really think this is going to make California more doable for you and Scott," she says, bringing out the big guns and hitting an important mark.

Relocating across the country for retransplant is a daunting stumbling block. It's my doctor's strong recommendation that, due to the sudden severity of my condition and the complexities of second transplants, I leave my home and my transplant hospital of twenty-six years (Columbia University Medical Center in New York) and head to Cedars-Sinai in Los Angeles for more specialized care. Waiting in California for a matching donor heart could take many months, and the recovery after transplant would add several more, making this a difficult and expensive undertaking. And all of my support—emotional and physical—would reside in Scott; isolated from family and friends, he would be the one keeping constant vigil day and night with no letup, all the while continuing to meet every one of the responsibilities of his job in New York. He'd worried aloud to me while imagining the multiple daily conference calls and long Skype meetings that would pull him away from my bedside even as I got sicker and needed him more. The pressure and stress on both of us would be enormous.

If I decided to go through with this, how would Scott and I manage? This question sank me under what seemed like an impossible weight.

Then Jill lifted it.

"I called the girls. We made a spreadsheet on Google Docs, see?" She brings up the image on her laptop and I move in for a closer look. "We've got you covered from mid-March through May. We'll fly out to California to be with you, one after the other. No gaps, see? And, of course, I'm comin' first."

How can this be? Every day . . . covered?

But I haven't even left yet . . .

My chin drops into my hand. I move my head from side to side as my eyes zoom in on the rectangles filled with the names of women from the tight-knit group we share. My closest friends had committed their most valuable gift in this moment of need: their unbroken chain of presence.

The sight of it sweeps me up—that within a simple spreadsheet, the depth of friendship could be laid bare like this. My throat tightens with tenderness as I gaze at the screen. Of all the women friend groups out there—in my town, in my state, in the world for that matter—*how many of them would actually do something like this . . . ?*

"Well, what do you think of it?" Jill asks, brown eyes searching mine. *Well.*

I thought it was quite a reveal. Quite a moment to remember. I felt my lips shoot up at the corners and set firmly in place—a snapshot of emotion. And then reality flashed, quick and terribly bright, and I wished to some God somewhere that my dying heart wasn't at the center of this picture.

"It's . . . it's . . . amazing. So wonderful of you. Of *everyone*. I don't know how to . . . to . . ."

"Thank us?" Jill takes my hand. "We love you, Ames. We want to do this for you."

I brush away a tear and take another look at the names of friends who've signed up so quickly—just like that. These women have school-age kids. Husbands. Jobs. Flying across the country to sit by my side will require significant juggling. It will also have my friends putting my needs before their long list of day-to-day responsibilities and commitments.

Am I worth that? Would I do the same for them—in an instant? It's the Scott question all over again: *When will I ever have the opportunity to do such an extraordinary act for each of these friends in return?*

Guilt rises up in me. My hands float instantly to the top of my head, where I begin to pull at strand after strand of hair, from scalp to end. Jill reaches out to lower my arms gently. "Who else d'you want?" She offers to contact anyone I might want to add to the schedule—friends from out of town or from law school, many of whom who she's never met.

"I'll call them tonight," she says, her eyes lighting up with pride in having orchestrated a tangible way to streamline my cross-country retransplant. "We are *there!*" she adds, snapping her laptop shut as if a deal has been sealed.

Then it hits me.

Wait.

Wait. Wait. Wait.

They are there. But am I?

What is happening here? The rush to the spreadsheet, while created out of genuine love and caring, feels like it is also Jill's way of speeding past my decision. As struck with emotion as I am upon seeing the little rectangles already filled in with friends' names, a sense of urgency rises in me to remind Jill that the swift commitment of these women may be all for nothing. My option to say no to retransplant must remain open, spreadsheet or not, and I can't help but hold tight to it with ferocity.

Jill knows this about me. So do Robin, Lauren, Val, and the others who've signed on. My friends have witnessed up close the havoc wreaked on my body from decades of transplant immunosuppressive medicines along with the declining function of my donor heart over time. They'd raced to my house when Scott was at work and I called them, frightened, "Can you please come sit with me? My pulse is one eighty, and it won't come down." They'd watched me swoon with nausea and weakness at dinner tables, and had missed me when I couldn't join them (yet again) on a group getaway because I had pneumonia or some other serious transplant-related infection. They'd heard me cry, "I can't do this anymore," and admitted to me in turn, "I couldn't do what you do every day."

And yet when it came to choosing between death and my continuing to do what they said they couldn't do, my friends would always stand with some percentage of a foot planted firmly in the camp of life. That firm stand taken by my friends, the one for me to fight for my life, diminished as they witnessed over the years what my transplant body put me through. We were probably down to mere toes by now, but I could still feel my friends' reservation against saying, finally, "Okay, Amy, *now* it's okay to just let go." And I understood their reluctance with the acuity and empathy that come from shared experience. After all, I was healthy once. I remembered well the innate and powerful drive toward living, the inability to imagine myself without breath, without movement. I couldn't even begin to contemplate choosing to end my days back then—not under any circumstance. Nothing could possibly be that bad, that unendurable.

The default for most everyone must always be life; it is perhaps the most powerful draw of all. Add to it a spreadsheet—a glittering mechanism of hope brought about by the dearest, most devoted friend, who cannot bear to think of my toes no longer beside hers in that camp of life—and I feel as if I might burst with love and appreciation.

And yet part of me wants to call every name on that list and confront them with the implications of what they're rallying around: my taking on additional trauma and suffering.

Looking at this spreadsheet, I find it difficult not to feel an imperative embedded in the dates and columns and boxes—that I choose re-transplant. From that comes the implied sense that whatever I have to endure going forward is not so bad as to make legitimate the question of whether to keep fighting for life. In some ways, this feels like an invalidation of all I've gone through over my twenty-five heart transplant years. And while I know this is not the overarching intent of Jill or any of the women on the spreadsheet, it nonetheless rushes to my very core and ignites a well-worn fuse of frustration that catches quick and explodes: *No one understands—no one fucking understands.*

A FEW DAYS later, I shoot off a provocative email to Jill without stopping to consider the ratio of passive to aggressive.

Within seconds, I feel my insides drop and twist: *That was shitty, Amy.*

The subject line reads, "This sounds like a great idea for me," and in the body of the email I've copied an article from the front page of the *New York Times* that Joy and I woke up to at my house just days before:

"'Aid in Dying' Movement Takes Hold in Some States."

"Helpful information!" I type in large font across the top. "The guy in the story has a deadly heart thing going on, like me. Looks like he can speed up his end and avoid additional suffering."

Jill doesn't answer. No friend can read an email like this and not back off, and I suppose it is what I intended. What I need is the time and space to focus on the most difficult choice I've ever had to make.

The New Mexico man featured in the article is grappling with an arduous decision as well: undergo complicated open-heart surgery or endure a painful cardiac death within a few months. He is adamant in refusing surgery because the open-heart aortic valve replacement he underwent recently was so brutalizing that he now prefers death to a repetition of such horror. He seeks the legal right to have a doctor help him avoid further torment and bring his life to a peaceful, dignified end before illness renders him too incapacitated to act. The article shows that several states, including New Mexico, are following in the wake of Oregon, which up until recently has been the only one to allow assisted dying. There is reason for this man to hope.

His particular medical situation gives me a new option to consider as well: if he is able to back out of life after one harsh surgery, then certainly I have double the justification to do the same right now, in anticipation of a second heart transplant. About eighteen months before the ominous breathlessness showed up in my bed at night, I too had undergone open-heart valve surgery just like the New Mexico man, but my valve repair had been performed on an enigmatic transplanted heart. A wayward maneuver of the razor-tipped catheter had sliced my tricuspid valve during a routine heart biopsy, causing a deadly leak. Surgery was the only option.

But transplanted hearts are seldom pried open and their valves mended with cuts and stitches years after original implantation; even my highly renowned valve surgeon had never taken on this unusual challenge. A few days before operating on me, he admitted freely to having limited knowledge, pushing back in his plush desk chair during our presurgery consultation and musing, "Not sure why, but I think there's something about tricuspid valve repair—a lot of fluid afterward." I imagined he was predicting waterlogged ankles or maybe a puffy belly for a while after surgery. But I learned the medical reality of what my surgeon had meant when, less than two days after the operation, simply taking in a breath would set off dagger stabs between my ribs. As it turned out, my lungs were drowning in a deluge of post-surgical fluid and there was no space for them to expand.

I would remember it mostly as agony and an abrupt midnight emergency invasion of sorts where a swarm of young doctors rushed to my bedside in the ICU, yanked me up to a sitting position, and thrust multiple stethoscopes toward my chest all at once. There were urgent orders—what seemed to be a team leader barking something about sterilizing the area and closing off doors so he could begin a surgical procedure right then and there at my bedside. I heard myself choking out words to one of the guys who wore scrubs and a bandana, "No mind-numbing drugs!" and then the admonition of a nurse looking me square in the eye and setting things straight: "You do not want to be awake for what they are about to do to you."

I allowed the drugs through my IV.

Sedation took me over. A doctor cut into the sides of my torso and drove thick tubes between my ribs and into both lungs to drain the fluid.

After that, my lungs were never the same. My heart wasn't either: in the year after the surgery, my tricuspid valve began leaking again (this time not severely enough to require surgery—yet). And even after a long, arduous recovery where I fought to return to presurgery strength, the only palpable improvement in my quality of life was the determination by my transplant cardiologist that heart biopsies were no longer safe for me. We would have to monitor rejection noninvasively. But even this victory was short-lived.

The symptoms that began three years ago on Casey's college move-in day have culminated—no longer cryptic now, but revealing their insidiousness with final clarity: my heart is succumbing to fatal failure, this time having nothing to do with my tricuspid valve, and my options are retransplant or die.

Or so it has seemed.

I learned during Joy's visit that there is a man in New Mexico who is fighting for the legal right to take advantage of a third option—a peaceful, painless, dignified death by choice, and boy, am I rooting for him.

I want Jill to know.

JOY AND I had just landed our spoons into cereal bowls when our eyes fell upon the article about assisted dying. Sitting side by side on high stools at my kitchen countertop table, we dove into the *New York Times* front page and read simultaneously, not speaking until we reached the last word.

"I can't believe this is the lead story today of all days," she said. We had planned to have breakfast and then spend hours by the fireplace talking through issues similar to those faced by patients in the article.

"No, no, I think the timing is perfect. I had no idea this kind of thing could be an option for heart patients. And look at this," I said, pointing to a few words on the continued interior page. "It's the name of the organization in Oregon—I've got to call there."

Joy shifted uncomfortably on her stool.

"Hmmm. Well . . . okaaay," she said, folding the paper slowly and pushing it across the countertop, away from us. I knew she was stalling, of course, trying to come up with a way to be supportive and stymieing at the same time. "We can include this in our options. But it's the weekend and they're probably closed today, right? And we need to know all the specifics, like what the residency requirements are. How you can get a doctor in Oregon or New Mexico or wherever . . ."

Delay, delay, delay.

There was no way Joy could abet or even abide my making a decision about assisted death on her watch, and while Scott was away.

"Let me just tell you this—Scott knows. It won't surprise him one bit if I reach out to Oregon for information before he gets home. He and I have talked many times about how I'm not going to keep up the good fight when the big one hits."

"But how do you know for sure this is the big one? And maybe you aren't even sick enough to qualify for assisted death."

"This *is* the big one, Joy. And you bet I am sick enough—and thank goodness for it. I am going to die unless I get a new heart. The Oregon option is a good one, Joy. And doable."

She sprang to standing. "More information, though. Lots more. Got to do this smart."

"Yeah, yeah, but we might as well call Oregon and see if they're open."

I grabbed a pen and skimmed the page again for the name of the organization. Out of the corner of my eye, I noticed that Joy had carried her bowl to the sink and stood with her back to me now, unmoving.

"You're upset," I said.

Joy turned around slowly. Her eyes were filled. "Look—this stuff you're saying to me isn't new, but it's still hard for me to hear because I love you, okay? And I know this is not about me, I really do. But I want you to live . . ." She tilted her head, shrugged, trying to be light. But then her shoulders came forward and shook with grief, and tears spilled down her face. "But that's just selfish me talking. What you've had to do just to survive all these years . . . it's beyond ridiculous. I think at this point, you've earned the right to decide not to go on."

I'd never heard this from a friend before—never.

"Thank you for saying that." I walked to the sink and reached my arms toward her. Joy had just voiced what I'd long wished all my friends could understand and confirm—that I had *earned* this decision. There was nothing I'd worked at harder or more diligently than the continued survival of my donor heart. And now I was exhausted from the years of transplant travails—and so was this heart; the poor thing was shutting down, bowing out, making it clear to all who listened through a stethoscope that it was done, never to rise up again.

But I'm supposed to keep rising, right?

"As much as it is possible to get it, I do—I get it," Joy said, midembrace, "and it's not just me—everyone will understand whatever you choose. Everyone supports you."

But this was where she was wrong. No one could ever see this situation as I did. Even back in 1988, when my doctor pegged my life expectancy at ten post-transplant years at best, my friends insisted on the greater wisdom of their own view. "Not *you*," they chided. "Heart transplant statistics haven't seen the likes of your amazing will and determination." Thereafter, they took every survival year as proof of my power over transplant realities.

But for every year survived I would implore them to remember the struggles—all the hospitalizations, the intractable infections, the skin cancers that kept coming back. And while they knew the litany of heart transplant scourges, everyone around me was swayed by the power of the other reality they saw: I was alive. It was hard for them to understand how I could view my end as I imagined my fading heart did now—*as a relief*. I had been waiting for my friends to soften their life stance so that I might soften mine too. But it was still a hot-button trigger for me every time someone broke into a recitation of *You're so strong, you have so much courage, what a superstar you are, is there nothing you can't survive, you're going to outlive all of us* . . .

Outlive all of us.

I had actually said that one aloud just a couple of weeks before Joy's visit—said it to the nurse whom I chose to be my *nice face* just moments after lying down on the angiogram table. "You warm enough?" she asked, covering me with a heated sheet. "Have to keep it real cold in here for the machines. But we're going to cover you with a whole mess of stuff in a minute. You'll be nice and snug under there." She wore a blue puffed surgical cap that matched her eyes. Her smile was young and easy. "I'm Sunny, by the way."

Of course you are. And you're going to be my nice face during the exam today—a pair of kind eyes across the room that I can count on for reassurance until this is over.

I needed to make a quick friend. "You know, Sunny, this is angiogram number twenty-eight for me."

"Is it now?" she said, unfurling a second layer of sterile draping from my feet to my neck. "Well, you must be an old pro."

"I guess so, but it never gets easier—the result, I mean. When the picture of my arteries comes up on the monitor, it's pretty scary. It's like a thumbs-up or thumbs-down moment in the Roman Colosseum."

She laughed, reaching up to retrieve the ceiling-mounted flat-screen monitor that would soon project my fate. "I never thought of it that way, but yes, it's a moment, and yours is going to be just fine today. Nice clean arteries. All those years bouncing around in ya—this heart's a keeper!"

I wouldn't be too sure, Sunny. You saw me hop up on this table when I came in here a few minutes ago, all spry and jaunty, with clear eyes, a strong voice, and looking as fit and healthy as any woman my age—you can't help but assume I am well.

But there was the nighttime breathlessness she knew nothing about; I was struggling for air even as I lay there chatting with her. And something even more ominous had been going on as well. "I've had pain down my arms for a few weeks now. Burning. Sometimes it's so bad I have to drop to the floor and roll around on the ground until it stops. My doctor says it's muscular, but I don't know."

She pressed a few buttons on the monitor, and it lit up in moving lines of yellows and greens. "Muscular, yeah, that's probably it. As I'm sure you know, there are no nerves attached to your heart, right? Surgeon cut those when they took out the one your mom and dad gave ya. Those nerves don't grow back."

I'd already learned this in the first year post-transplant, but I didn't want to say that. I needed to hear Sunny's voice right now, and her attribution of my discomfort to muscle strain gave me a little boost of hope. After all, Sunny was a nurse in a catheterization lab (or cath lab), which specialized in using catheters to help visualize the arteries and chambers of the heart. She would know the symptoms of clogged arteries.

With a flick of her wrist in the air, she tried to wave off my worry. "You transplant patients can't feel any cardiac pain even if you're havin' it. Maybe you're just overdoing it when you exercise. Ever try taking a bath in Epsom—"

"No. I feel it at rest too. When I am just sitting there."

"Hmmm," she said, pursing her lips.

A tech broke the silence: "Here's Dr. Romani. Let's get going." I watched Sunny move behind the X-ray shield that would become a barrier between us until the exam was over. She fastened a surgical mask to cover her mouth and nose, but I could still see her eyes.

"No sedation, please, like always, Dr. Romani," I said.

"Yes, dear, I know," he answered flatly. After two decades of angiograms with this guy, he still did not know my name. But he remembered that I was the rare patient who insisted on doing these exams fully awake; sedation was the usual protocol, and most people on the angiogram table were more than happy to sleep through its challenges.

I wasn't. For me, every invasive exam or procedure was an opportunity to increase my capacity for abidance and courage—skills I would have to call on constantly in my life with a heart transplant. If I could bear the onslaught of physical challenges on the cath lab table—the needle sticks, the slices into my skin, the feeling of catheters snaking up through my torso—then I might better tolerate and push through the nausea and general flu-like symptoms that were daily side effects of my transplant medicines. And if I could manage to direct my mind into a reasonably calm state without chemically concealing what I physically endured during each invasive procedure, then bravery might sooner become a reliable asset in my day-to-day life. What doesn't kill you makes you stronger, indeed.

"Since you're not sedated, you are going to feel this. Sorry about that," Dr. Romani said.

"Yup, I know the drill. Just do your thing."

"Okay, let's begin. Cold and wet." This meant he was applying sterile solution to clean a shaven spot on the left side of my groin. Lying prone, I couldn't see his moves, but I knew each of them in sequence by rote.

"And now some numbing medicine," I said, before he did.

An injection of lidocaine. And another. And then another.

"Ouch, ouch, ouch," I squeaked.

"Sorry, dear. Are you all right?"

"I'm fine. It hurts, but this part is never the hard part for me. It's the pictures. I want my arteries to look like they did last time."

Last time had been four months ago, during a scheduled annual checkup. The results had been fine (unchanged from previous exams, that is), so I was not supposed to have another angiogram for a year. Today's was an emergency add-on.

"We'll get a good look and see," the doctor said. "Big push, aaaand . . . we're good."

With the artery plug now in place, Dr. Romani began threading the body-length catheter through the slit he'd cut my groin, moving it up into my heart; once there, he would push dye through and take X-ray images as the dark liquid filled my arteries with prognostic shading. Solid black trunks, branches, and branchlets, like those of sturdy trees in wintertime, were good. Bits of lighter gray dispersed along their outlines or, worse, concentrated into a section that appeared to narrow their width or divide them into distinct segments—well . . .

It was time to find Sunny's eyes. They were directed toward the screen, awaiting the first image.

A whir of machinery signaled the start-up of the X-ray apparatus suspended like a giant crane above my forehead, its flat radiating disk the size of a large pizza. Down, down it slid, just nearly skimming my nose, chin, and upper chest—until it came to rest directly over my heart.

"Fluoro!" the doctor called out, alerting the room to the radiation now flowing from this souped-up X-ray they called a fluoroscope.

"Sunny, I need your nice face. This is the part I hate. I should just be optimistic, yeah, I've done this so many times and everything has been okay. Why should my heart go bad now? You know what my doctor said—he said maybe at almost twenty-six years after transplant, I'm home free. No transplant artery disease for me—not ever, right? I'm going to be an old, old lady one day. Who knows? My friend Deirdre, she tells me all the time, 'You're going to outlive all of us,' so maybe she is right, or maybe . . . well, we will see in a minute, won't we . . ."

Intense fear had me babbling even though I sensed I was talking to no one; Sunny did not seem to be listening anymore.

I felt the dye making its way through my veins like warm honey.

"I really, really need your face."

"Here I am," Sunny said cheerfully, and shifted her eyes to meet mine for only for a split second. A masked face without eyes was going to do me no good now.

"Okay, here's a poem I memorized for today." I knew I could have recited it silently to myself, but I had to try to feel connected somehow with the people in the room—lab techs, doctor, resident, two nurses—even though they stood apart from me, masked, behind X-ray-proof screens. I had only myself to turn to—no Scott, no friend, no nice face. The aloneness was torture in that moment, just as it had been at all my angiograms, heart biopsies, surgeries, and midnight rescues in the ICU—the kind of terrified isolation that comes when you feel the edge of the guillotine blade against your neck, I imagined. Those who love you may weep and wail, distraught over the thought of losing you. But the most unthinkable loss was your own: you were going lose yourself.

"'I Wandered Lonely as a Cloud,' by William Wordsworth. *I wandered lonely as a cloud that floats on high o'er vales and hills, when all at once I saw a crowd . . .*"

Up came the first image, followed quickly by the second. Moving my gaze clockwise, I noted a big black trunk and branch, another big black branch, smaller branchlets with—what was that, gray? I turned my head to look at Sunny, who continued to focus on the screen; I saw no reaction and told myself, *All right, then, it can't be too bad.* I took a deep breath and exhaled, readying myself for the next two pictures to come. Memory told me there should be about four in total.

Dr. Romani injected more dye. Again, the honey veins.

"*. . . a host, of golden daffodils; beside the lake, beneath the trees, fluttering and dancing in the . . .*"

Third image and then the fourth: solid black trunk, some dark gray, and then lighter, fading out into—*uh-oh*—wispy branchlets so narrow I could hardly—*oh God*—

"Sunny?"

There she was, repositioned at a stainless steel countertop at the far end of the room. She lifted her hand as if to say, *Request noted,* and set to jotting intently in what looked like a ledger book.

Rather than be angry with her, I felt sorry. Sunny had been so upbeat, so positive, but my healthy appearance and medical chart full of excellent cholesterol numbers and transplant longevity had thrown her off. It would be hard for her to stand beside me now and say, *Whoops.*

"What did you see, Dr. Romani?" In my other exams, he would have said *Looks good* by now. But what I just saw on the screen was something else entirely.

He stepped away from the table and nodded to a tech whose job it was to remove the plug from my groin and apply pressure until the bleeding stopped. "I don't know transplanted hearts. You're going to have to wait to speak with Dr. Davis."

"Since when don't you know transplanted hearts? What's *that* all about? Please just tell me what you see. Are there changes?"

"One area looks, um, different from last time. There is some progression. I don't know what that means for you exactly. Your doctor will tell you what to do about it."

"Progression—that's bad," I said, welling with tears.

A small area of plaque had shown up in one of my arteries during my eighth post-transplant year, but Dr. Romani had reassured me after every angiogram since then that the pictures looked pretty much the same. Stable plaque was unremarkable. Any increase, I knew, could be a sign of creeping vasculopathy.

"Let's get you cleaned up and out of here. Are you in any pain, dear?"

"P-pain? N-n-no." My teeth started chattering. I pressed my lips together and tried to reset my composure. "No pain. But tell me this: I've got vasculopathy, right? The thing that kills transplant patients. Small vessels in my heart are full of g-gray—I s-saw it . . ." The chattering again. Panic overtook me. I balled my hands into fists and thrust them up and up again to slacken the tightly tucked sheets that pinned my arms against my sides. With a few shoulder shrugs, I was able to pull up my elbows and then, *whoop*, my arms were free and waving above me, grazing the fluoroscope. I was desperate to escape now—bolt from the room, race down the hall, call out to Scott . . .

Dr. Romani turned his back to me and started for the door. "I'll go let your husband know that we're all done and that Dr. Davis will be speaking with you both soon," he said, abandoning me to the playing out of a nightmare moment I had dreaded for nearly twenty-six years. It had come true just as I had imagined—

Look up at the screen. See arteries filled with transplant disease. Know that this is the end of my heart. I am going to die soon, and no one is talking to me. There is no hand to hold. Only a masked tech standing beside the exam table, pressing a wad of gauze against my groin for five minutes, ten, fifteen, until the hole in my artery dries up sufficiently to roll me into the recovery area on a stretcher. And I lie there until a nurse deems it is safe for Scott to come in.

"Can I use my cell phone?" I asked the tech. I had taken it with me into the catheterization lab and had pushed it under my butt cheek before the sterile draping piled on.

"Okay, but keep your hips and legs real still."

I slid the phone out from under me and dialed Jill at the office. She was always my first call after every angiogram and had listened intently to my blow-by-blow recitations of what happened each year on the exam table. The words *some progression* would frighten her as they did me.

One ring. Two . . .

I hung up.

No. I can't speak to her right now.

Recognizing immediately that things were bad, Jill was going to ask what could be done about this test result. I would have to tell her that, as far as I know, there was really only one way to survive serious vasculopathy: another heart transplant.

And she would expect me to do it. Everyone would.

You're the Energizer Bunny, a survivor, a warrior, you can get another twenty-six years out of a heart, hell, we'll be in our seventies—but you, Wonder Woman, you'll probably keep going and . . .

Outlive you all?

Every friend, every family member, even my doctors were invested in the belief that longevity was everything, but that was their goal, not mine. I wanted to live long, sure, and I loved my donor heart—it had carried me, against all odds, through graduate school and on to many years of marriage and motherhood and friendship. I was so grateful for it that I worked with near compulsive diligence to keep it free from rejection and transplant vasculopathy—consuming not a sip of alcohol or pat of butter in almost twenty-six years, jogging and jogging no matter how sick I felt as I ticked off the miles, and swallowing the required immune-system-squelching, cancer-causing pills every day without fail for almost three decades. I treasured my precious donor heart so much I even allowed my doctor to biopsy it to destruction without question.

But the cost had been heavier than that. The cost was loneliness.

And I was alone in my resolve that choosing death must always be a real option for me. I knew that at some point, a medical horror would come along and combine with all the others before it, and I would say to everyone around me as calmly as I could, "This is where I stop. I will fight no more body battles."

"We'll see," was what I heard most often in response. My determination to set limits on the fight for life did not make sense to normal, healthy people. It didn't even fit with the outlook of most sick people. But mine was a credo that grew and strengthened as the decades of extreme heart transplant survival efforts chipped away at me: ambulance rides late at night, dozens of hospitalizations and close-call emergency interventions, nearly one thousand doctor visits, and well over one hundred invasive tests and procedures. Even so, this credo was an unfathomable belief to others, one that prompted the people I love and respect to say to me, "This is just not something I can support."

But I needed the people I loved to hear it anyway, if only as preparation; I knew that someday there would be those deathly blockages of gray up on the angiogram monitor. So I had made a point of sharing with each of my friends a conversation I'd had with Scott on a mountaintop.

He and I had been standing on a high perch in the Tetons overlooking a shimmering lake when I found opportunity in the beautiful view. "There's something I want you to know," I said, turning suddenly serious. "You see me here today—I couldn't be happier or more clearheaded. So, please, take me seriously now when I tell you I love life and I adore you, but at some point, it's going to be one too many god-awful transplant horrors and I may decide not to fight—enough will be enough. And when that time comes, please don't think I'm not in my right mind, because I'm saying this to you right now and it's not emotion talking."

It was not the first time I'd told Scott what I would and would not agree to do medically, but most often it had been under the duress of acute illness. This particular day in the mountains gave me a chance to make a definitive statement set against a background of perfect calm and happiness. There could be no discounting my words by saying, *You're just upset.*

But when he looked at me way up there, framed against a cobalt sky at ten thousand feet, my hair in a long, low braid, thick pink socks peeking out the top of dusty hiking boots, backpack with half-empty water bottles and what was left of our homemade trail mix, there was no way that my great love, my Scott, could imagine me choosing to say good-bye to life—or to him.

He looked out into the distance, taking in the sweeping view. "Yeah, all right, okay," he said.

And we continued our climb.

I TURN ON the small lamp beside my bed and reach for the notebook in my night table drawer—quiet, quiet, I don't want to wake Scott, who's just returned from his business trip, exhausted. Sticking out from the top of the pages is a piece of yellow paper folded vertically down the middle. On the left is a string of sentences I copied down carefully from their original source.

Shakespeare. A soliloquy.

I chose this particular one for memorization just after the ominous burning pain started in my arms and chin several weeks ago. Some scribbles on the right half of the page remind me that I've already set to my routine of writing the words from memory again and again, as best I can. There are errors; I haven't gotten it perfect yet. I pick up a pencil and try anew.

To be or not to be, that is the question . . .

Holy crap, yes. That is exactly the question.

And just today, finally, one month after glimpsing my heart's doom on the angiogram screen, I found my answer. It wasn't Jill's spreadsheet that delivered me to it. It wasn't Scott's return from his trip that tipped the scale either—our long embrace at the door or the adoring wonder in his voice as he pulled back for a moment and took in the sight of me in my flannel pajamas, saying, "How can you still look so darn adorable with all that's going on?"

No—what did it was this: I lost my breath while retrieving the mail from the bottom of my driveway this morning, and it frightened the hell out of me. I had to stop midway up the small slope, about thirty feet short of my house. It was raining ice, and I thought I might collapse right there, fall to the gravel, and freeze.

Scott will be the first to find me when he gets home from his trip tonight.

I wished I'd thought to take a cell phone with me.

I have to carry my cell to the mailbox now. Has it come to this already?

The deterioration of my heart function was speeding up, just as my doctor had said it would.

I have to get inside. I have to make it there.

I lowered myself to the ground—bare hands and denim-covered knees against frozen slush—and I crawled.

Breathe breathe breathe breathe . . .

This gasping was different from what I'd fought in bed each night.

Instead of heaviness in my chest, I felt alarmingly light. Empty. My lungs were flaccid balloons poked with holes. The feeling was all lack. Incapacity. The loss of breath's effect.

The feeling was death, and it was unbearable.

I reached the garage and inched my back along its grooved surface until I stood on two feet again. And there it was in the perspective and gratitude that came of terror relieved: my answer. I would not choose to just let my body come to its end—by assisted suicide or otherwise. I would say yes to retransplant.

As strong as I had been in my determination not to fight on when the big one hit, I wasn't nearly brave or mighty enough to watch myself actually suffocate. The time had come when the desperate practice of breathing into windowpanes seemed quaint; crawling on ice had shown me a new reality.

Thus conscience does make cowards of us all . . .

Shakespeare's words.

Returning to the page in front of me, I prop myself taller against my pillow and write them from memory now. I've made it nearly to the end of the soliloquy and stop here.

Okay, so I'm a coward. Now what?

Travel arrangements, packing for five months, transfer of hospital records, looking online for a rental near the hospital . . .

Jill's spreadsheet. For the first time, it makes me smile.

It strikes me that there's more for me in her creation than she realizes. There's an opportunity for meaningful time with my best friends, and with that there's also a chance to be understood. My closest friends would bear witness to the realities and complexities of surviving so long with a transplanted heart—and perhaps I could emerge from onerous expectations, able to show everyone without having to explain myself: *This is what I live, this is what I have lived.*

How lonely I have felt over these decades of illness, hidden in plain sight—even from those I love—appearing on the outside like most any other woman, but churning so differently on the inside. What a relief it would be to have friends join me, finally, in the full light of truth.

And if I die out there in California with these women at my side, well, I will die understood. Of the many factors that drive my decision to go for retransplant, Jill has hit on this one unknowingly.

I sent that email to her yesterday to say that I still believe in options. This New Mexico man makes great sense to me and I agree with his right to choose his end.

But I am going to California . . .

3

---

kay, I'll give you to Mom now," Scott says, handing me his
cell phone.

I take it and smile as if my son could see me. "Hi, Casey-
boy, what's up today?" There's no need to repeat what Scott already told
him: that our takeoff was delayed due to wind and snow in New York,
but we're in LA safe and sound, unpacking, and our little rental bunga-
low is great—just two blocks from the hospital!

"Tired." Casey sighs through a big yawn. It's one p.m. on Sunday
and he's just getting up.

"Late night?"

"Yeah, and I've got a ton of work to do."

"Heading out to the library, then?"

"We're going out for breakfast first."

Muffled giggles in the background; he's got a girl with him. "Well,
I won't keep you . . ."

"Yeah. Listen, Mom, I need you to, uh . . . I'm running low on heavy
socks."

I tell him I'll ask a friend to grab a few pairs at the house and mail them. "Love you," I say, and hand the phone back to Scott. He walks quickly from the room while continuing the conversation, his voice trailing off as he steps out onto the front porch. "And Casey, you should really think about coming out here for your March break . . ."

It's February, and we last saw him at New Year's. We haven't spoken to him much in the intervening time; Casey is an independent sort who calls only occasionally and sends a few texts a week.

"Did you tell him I'm worse?" I ask Scott when he returns to the bedroom to help store the empty suitcases in the back of the closet.

"No."

"Good."

He sits on the bed, flops himself back, and looks at the ceiling. "Yeah, I guess . . ."

"You don't think we should ask him to come here right away, do you?"

My question lands us in the same tough spot we found ourselves a few weeks ago when the bad-news angiogram back in New York sparked an immediate discussion about whether to bring Casey home. But neither one of us saw any use in interrupting the start-up of the second semester of his junior year; Casey would fly in from Oberlin and—what? Watch us cry? Listen in as I deliberated whether I'd go for a second heart transplant or not? Watch sad friends arrive in our living room, one after the next? We would never allow it.

Scott and I devoted ourselves to keeping my health worries as far from Casey's sight as possible during his childhood and teen years. It took some fancy footwork on both our parts: a lot of formulated cheerfulness through scary times; a lot of hiding how sick I felt when showing up for soccer games, music recitals, and sleepover pickups; a lot of Scott's nuancing of the truth—*Yeah, Mom's in the hospital for a few days, nothing serious, just her usual tests.* Most of our teamwork was seamless and successful, a coordinated sleight of hand to keep Casey distracted with kid stuff while I eked out daily survival as inconspicuously as possible.

But this time it's different. This time there is a good chance I won't make it. And Casey is almost twenty-one now; Scott and I agree that we should start talking with him more openly and honestly about my health. Even so, we don't want to turn his college life upside down unless and until we have no other choice.

"Let's stick with our plan—no plucking him out of school," Scott says, definitively. "He'll come to LA during his break next month. And meanwhile, I really think you should write him a letter that I can hold onto just in case."

"A letter. You mean, like . . . a final good-bye. In writing."

He nods.

I lower myself beside him on the bed and exhale, hand to chest. "I *can't*."

"I know it's hard, but you have to. You're his mother. He's going to need some words from you . . ."

"Of course, yes, sure. I just don't . . . How do I . . ."

He places two fingers under my chin and lifts it gently so our eyes are in line. "Just tell him you love him. You'll find the words. But you need to do it and you need to do it soon."

I assure him I will, I will.

A few days later, I sit down at the makeshift dining room table with a piece of white copy paper and a plain envelope pulled from the small stash we brought with us from home, and I give it a try:

Dear Caseyboy,

I love you so and I'm terribly sorry I am not with you anymore. But how lucky I am to have been your mom for all these years—to hold little tiny you in my arms, to watch you grow, to be there for you when . . .

I put my pen down. No mother should have to do this.

I drop my head into my hands. A wave of foreboding crashes over me: that if my fight for life is unsuccessful and this letter transfers into Casey's possession, he will feel that I have failed him.

But, Casey, don't you see? I eked out almost twenty-six years with a heart slated for something like ten. It was an amazing feat, my son. And I never once told you how difficult—

I don't have it in me. I just don't have it in me . . .

I wipe my eyes and keep going.

RECLINING ON A chaise in the tiny front garden of our bungalow, I feel a peck, quick but sure, at the side of my right hand. A tiny glistening shape springs vertically. I turn my head to follow, and there it is: a hummingbird. It shoots over to a wiry little tree, lands for a second, and whirs to a fence post before zooming straight for the bougainvillea in full magenta bloom.

"Leja! Come here!" I call out to my friend, who is sitting on the porch rocker, reading.

She jumps, throws aside her *People* magazine, and dashes down the three steps from house to garden, her ice-blue eyes wide with fear. "What is happened! What you need me!"

"No, no, I'm fine. Sorry. I didn't mean to scare you. Just this second—it was wild!—a hummingbird flew from the tree and pecked me with its beak. Look! He's still in the flowers there!"

"What! Does it hurt to you!" Her hands splay out and land on her chest.

"Not at all, Leja, calm down. Do you see him? Wait, I think he flew away . . ."

She slaps her palm against her forehead. "Whew, okay, okay. I am so scary. I thought you were of a sudden . . ."

Leja is on edge, and understandably so. She arrived here just yesterday and is the first friend to join us at the bungalow. Scott and I aren't quite sure how to fit her in; we haven't yet let go of the rhythm we've fallen into over the past week here alone. Suddenly we are three, and as

we knew would be the case with Leja, our new addition is a conspicu-
ous and skittish presence.

She pivots away and kicks at some pebbles near the flower bed.

"We're going to have to figure out how to do this," I say.

"Do what?"

"You know. Take care of me without taking care of me."

"It is okay to me," she says softly, but I know that these words—
spoken in her Eastern European syntax—don't mean what they would
in plain English: that she is happy to take care of me however I wish.
No, Leja is saying something much kinder and deeper, something that
goes back nearly twenty years to the first day she showed up at my
bedside with a blue plastic bucket in one hand and a mop in the other,
asking, "Where you would like that I start?"

All those years ago, an infection had landed me in bed while Scott
was in China on business for two weeks. Joy had planned to visit for
the weekend anyway, so she flew in from DC and subbed in for me—
cooking, cleaning, and shuttling Casey to friends' houses, sports
games, ice-skating. After twenty-four hours, she insisted, "You are go-
ing to get live-in help—at least for the winter months when you're sick
like this all the time." A few days later I found Leja through a classified
ad and hired her on the spot.

"Please start anywhere downstairs," I said, barely able to lift my
head to speak, "and I'm sorry I can't get up to show you around today.
I'm not usually this sick. I'm actually quite strong and I like to clean
the house myself . . ."

She looked at me with owl eyes, unblinking.

"No, really. I'm fine. Just not today."

"Okay," she said, reaching down for a pair of rubber gloves at the
bottom of the bucket and coming up again to meet my eyes directly.
"It is okay to me." What she actually meant by this was: *It is a feeling I
know too.*

Leja has an intense will to effect change in spite of impossibility, and
she sensed the same in me immediately. Within a few weeks I would

come to recognize in her a few additional sensibilities and hard-earned traits we shared. The brazen honesty. The powerful self-discipline. The sheer grit it takes to keep suiting up in full armor to meet the challenges of our respective lives, clenching our jaws with determination to make our days better, easier, more like those of other women we see around us—and yet knowing that our efforts will either fall far short of our dreams, or fail.

It is this shared reality that made it possible for me to say in just a few months of knowing her that she was one of my closest friends. Up until the time Leja's six-month visa expired, necessitating her return to Croatia, she and I put in more hours of face-to-face discussion, pointed debate, and unabashed belly laughter than I had with all my other friends combined. And when there were tears—bitter, streaming ones as we feared for each of our futures—we shared whatever armor we had, promising our presence and protection to each other now and always. So, when Leja returned to America for short, visa-sanctioned stints in the years that followed, I welcomed her without hesitation to live at my house while she worked in nearby towns. And this strengthened our bond even more: we grew from our thirties to our forties together, talking long and late at the kitchen table and relying on our deep understanding and interdependence to carry us through the unfixable frustrations and challenges of our respective days.

I look up at my dear Leja on the porch rocker now; she's been keeping me company from a distance, which is perfect, but I only just noticed this for the first time all afternoon. Turns out, she started figuring how best to be with me in this California setup even before I told her we needed to work on it.

I soften and reach out. "What're you readin' in your *People* magazine over there?"

She holds up the cover so I can see the headline: "Too Thin Too Fast."

"Ha! I know, I know, you think that's not possible—*too thin*—but, ah, never mind . . ." I learned years ago that the best way to deal with

Leja's nutty penchant for leanness is with lighthearted humor. I trill a few *cuckoo-cuckoo*s, and she waves me off once with the back of her hand.

"Look at this one here . . ." She flips to an inside page and turns it in my direction. It's a photograph of an athletic woman whom I can't identify—probably a popular, young actress. "She is, I think, a little fa-a-at."

For Leja, fat is one syllable spoken in three long beats.

"Like I am, you mean?"

"Nooo," she says with an extra-wide grin, perhaps recalling our run-in years earlier when she told me, "You are fat, like Angelina Jolly," after she'd tried on a pair of jeans that no longer fit me. Leja's matchstick legs swam in excess. Taking the pants off, she wondered aloud if maybe they might fit her cousin back in Croatia because she was my size (size two).

I swatted Leja's rear end with a wire hanger that day. "I am not fat, and neither is Angelina *Jolie*, but okay, I will say what I know you want to hear—yes, Leja, you are definitely skinnier than me."

"I know!" she squealed, gleeful as she pivoted sideways to check out her utter flatness in the mirror behind my closet door. Reaching up with both hands, Leja swept her long black hair into a quick topknot, put some sexy fire into her wide-set eyes, and smiled devilishly. "And I love it!"

But here on the porch today, Leja is more serious. She closes the magazine and slaps her hand on the cover. "Well! I say these woman are not skinny to me!"

"All rightie."

There was no changing her mind—Leja believed what she believed and stated her views without apology. And I admired her confidence, the way she lifted her chin and spoke the truth of things as she saw it, no matter how unusual or objectionable to people around her.

All reasons why I have come to call her my Croatian sister.

Leja pops up from the rocker as a burst of energy overtakes her.

"Now I will look for this bird!" She darts here and there in the garden, swatting at the sky and squinting into the sun in search of a hummingbird flown. She will not let up, I know, until she gets a sighting. "Come back, come back! Where you are?" she calls.

"It's gone. Why don't you come sit," I offer gently and pull up my knees to make room at the end of the chaise. She makes a few more traverses, freezes midstep, and lowers herself to the chaise cushion slowly, absently. I know the meaning of her momentary trancelike state; I have seen it before when Leja's racing mind starts weaving a tale of significance out of something. This time it is a peck from a bird's beak, and she lets its import seep in like tattoo ink until her conviction becomes indelible. I ready myself for something Leja-esque.

"This hummingbird. Maybe he is a sign," she tells me, crouching into a forward lean as if she were about to tell a ghost story. She brings her voice down to a breathy whisper: "Birds are signs. They carry messages. One time, a bird landed on the hood of my car and would not go. Wings move like this"—she shows me, flapping her arms exaggeratedly—"and next day, my brother called from Croatia to say to me that my uncle, he died. This hummingbird tells to you something. What did you notice from him?"

I'd like to stop this right here. Getting up from the chaise every few minutes to catch my breath, I can't put much thought into a hummingbird—no matter how laden with portent. But Leja can't help but get revved up with curiosity, just as she does for all happenings big and small, especially when there is something new or different to tempt her excitability. I've seen this when I return from an outing with Scott, be it a hike up north or a day in New York City: Leja will plant herself in my kitchen and demand endless details. Looking through my photographs, she will point out a flower—"What the name is?"—and cluck at me when I don't know. "You are in this place and it shows to you beautiful flowers, and you do not care!" she scolds. And after a visit to the Museum of Modern Art? Leja will be waiting for me at day's end, wanting to know not only if I saw the Picassos but also "Which they are, the paintings?" and whether I listened to the headset for a full description of each. If I admit to her that I skipped a few, she becomes incredulous. "Oh, if I could to be there, I would listen every one!"

Most days, I love this about Leja: the way she dives into minute details, thrilling at things I would otherwise give short shrift. But for me, every day here in California is about waiting for a phone call from my new transplant team at Cedars-Sinai that a donor match has come through, and hoping that my worsening symptoms will not pluck me from this bungalow and land my time bomb heart in a hospital before the call comes.

I look through the screen door and see Scott inside; he's supposed to be working at the dining room table, but instead he paces anxiously. "It's not going to happen just yet, honey," I whispered late last night when I woke to find him sitting up in bed with the light on, staring out at nothing. He understood that my high levels of antibodies meant that Cedars would likely not be calling me soon with news of a matching donor heart, and it frightened him. I was getting weaker by the day, unable to walk the blocks I had managed when we first arrived two weeks earlier. Unable now to sit at the table for meals. Showering quicker or not at all because the physical demands of soaping up and rinsing myself robbed me of oxygen. Even without my calling his attention to these signs of worsening heart failure, Scott noticed them. Leja did too, I could be sure of it, with her sharp, observant eye that knew my habits well. But she remained her enthusiastic, energetic self, eager to keep my mind off the waiting any way she could. Yesterday it was her overflowing love for palm trees, the first she had ever seen in her forty-five years. Today it is distraction by hummingbird.

I really should oblige her with an answer. "Well . . . the bird, he seemed, um, happy, I guess."

"Happy. Very good! And what sign to you it is?"

"All right, all right. Let me think for a minute," I say, but I am only pretending to ponder. A hummingbird connection occurred to me the minute I saw the tiny blue-green shape dart from chaise to fence post;

I just don't feel like getting into it with Leja, who would surely bubble over. I see, though, that she will not let this pass; I am going to have to get this over with and give her a response to chew on.

"Wait a minute . . . there *is* something about hummingbirds actually," I say. "You know what *essay* means, yes, a piece of writing on a subject? Okay, so there's this essay about hummingbirds that I read a couple of years ago in a literary journal—a little book with articles inside, you know what I mean?"

She nods.

The essay actually was as much about hummingbirds as it was about hearts, which was why it grabbed my attention. I downloaded the piece in its entirety and sent it to my cardiologist on the twenty-fifth anniversary of my transplant.

"Seems I am a hummingbird," I wrote to him. "Read this and you'll see—there I am!"

"Consider the hummingbird for a long moment," the essay began. "A hummingbird's heart beats ten times a second . . . the most amazing thing you have never seen, each thunderous wild heart the size of an infant's fingernail . . ."

The beating within my chest was thunderous as well. And wild. From the time it took up residence beneath my breastbone, the heart I received from my thirteen-year-old donor revved like a race car. Even at complete rest, my pulse would drive hard at 115 beats per minute. The slightest bit of exercise—pulling a load of towels out of the dryer, carrying a bag of groceries into the house—would send it soaring to a quick 160. I complained to my doctor about it a few months after transplant, and he dismissed it. "Your heart is not attached to your central nervous system anymore. With all the nerves cut and gone, your heart can't receive a signal telling it to slow down or speed up. Plus, your donor, she was very young. Teenage hearts tend to beat faster." This meant that I would always sense my denervated heart, as doctors called it, being propelled not by body intelligence, but rather by adrenaline—the new and unruly source of my willy-nilly pulse rate.

It would take some getting used to, my doctor warned. But I never would get used to it. No matter how relaxed I was, my heart would race. After a few years living this way, I forgot what it felt like to be completely at ease. My whole sense of being had been forever altered at twenty-five.

Only after reading an essay decades later did I realize that my transplanted heart had transformed me into a hummingbird. And now one of these amazing creatures had found its way to my little bungalow in West Hollywood—with intent to touch my hand, perhaps?

Leja would see it this way.

"I remember the essay talked about how hummingbirds have to fly so fast, all over the place to get nectar, their food, you know?" I say, causing her to launch both hands toward her mouth in anticipation. She bites at her fists. "They have to land on something like a thousand flowers a day to get the food energy they need. So their hearts are like airplane engines, powerful, zipping them all sorts of ways—straight up, backwards. Hummingbird hearts are a wonder . . . and when you think about it, they're like my heart, right? Unusual and kind of unbelievable."

Leja breaks into a full smile of sparkling white teeth. "This is a sign! We are in California. The hospital is two blocks to us. You are sit and wait for a new heart." She grabs my knees. "What this bird tells to you—you will get a heart soon!"

But this would be almost impossible. Even though I'd reviewed some basic heart transplant science and how the system works with Leja and other friends before heading out here, it was still hard for them to understand why optimism about my chances on the Cedars waiting list made no sense. I tried to tell them in simple terms that even if I were at the top of the list (and I was not quite sick enough for that yet), the likelihood of finding a matching heart would still be extremely low. My friends heard this as negativity and yet another excuse for waffling on my decision for retransplant. As they saw it, since I got a heart almost twenty-six years ago, I would get one again. But science had changed over this long stretch of time, and so had my body.

Unlike back in 1988, when heart transplant science was nascent and donor hearts were paired with recipients based merely on blood type and size, the modern approach prescreens donor-recipient matches by using a sophisticated gene-based analysis of antibodies in the blood. Closer matches mean fewer rejection episodes going forward, a decrease in the incidence of early vasculopathy, and longer survival rates in some cases. But in a select few patients, a high number of antibodies (including specific ones that are especially dangerous) can stand as a barrier to successful transplant. I am one of those cases.

Living with a foreign heart for nearly three decades (sadly, a donor heart will always be seen by the body's immune system as foreign), I have amassed a number of particularly malicious antibodies. Adding to this were the blood transfusions I've had over my transplant years due to the valve repair and other surgeries; donated blood also remains forever foreign to its recipient. Friends heard these facts and still did not let it dampen their outlook on my chances, even though I had hard numbers to show them. Their optimism had been buoyed by the unreliability of numbers for decades now, tallying up my post-transplant years with increasing breeziness as I moved further and further beyond the ten-year life expectancy pronounced by my doctors early on. Optimistic ovations like *You're an odds-beater* roll easily off their tongues, along with *You leave doctors scratching their heads every time.* And my friends are right: I've had several cardiologists call me an *"n* of one" as they applied fingernails to scalp—scratch, scratch.

But there is no medical mystery in the effect of antibodies on transplanted hearts. Interpretation requires no conjecture—only the application of science. And the science, in my case, is unequivocal.

After last month's angiogram revealed that my heart is riddled with vasculopathy, my transplant cardiologist at Columbia, Dr. Davis, ordered an antibody blood analysis. The results were stupefying: sky-high antibodies, including the dreaded, virulent C1q—a marker known to be lethal to any donor heart. The combination of excessive quantity and dangerous quality of antibodies circulating in my body slashed the potential donor population from which I could receive a heart to only 14 percent. Or, looked at another way, between the shortage of donor hearts and the fact that I would be incompatible with 86 percent of the donor pool, the odds are stacked against me.

"You won't make it here in New York," Dr. Davis told me when I sat across his desk to discuss next steps. "California is the only real option." Given the inauspicious results on my antibody blood panel and the extensive waiting list at Columbia, it was unlikely that I would get a donor heart in my home state before a year and a half. My heart did not have that kind of time. He put aside the antibody issue for a moment, explaining first that Cedars-Sinai in California receives more donor hearts than Columbia because of the way organs are allocated according to the United Network for Organ Sharing.

This did not surprise me. In earlier years, I'd served on the board of UNOS—the federally contracted body that governs transplant waiting lists and organ donation/procurement. Under UNOS regulations, a highly defined grid delineates the areas from which transplant hospitals in each state can have first dibs at an organ for transplant. When I first saw the UNOS map of organ procurement regions, I located my home state and noticed that it seemed to be at a disadvantage. New York is in Region 9, along with western Vermont; this means a donor heart that becomes available in one of these two states will first be offered locally (i.e., within this region). I soon learned that New York is not known for robust organ donation, and Vermont's population is just too small to serve the high demand of the two-state region. It didn't seem fair.

When Dr. Davis recommended I go to Cedars-Sinai, I pulled out my old UNOS map and took a close look at the West Coast. California is in Region 5, which it shares with Utah, Arizona, New Mexico, and Nevada. Five states. Not a large number of transplant centers within them. And, as I remembered hearing at UNOS board meetings, a kinder California has a more generous donor pool, for reasons I never came to understand.

But, as my doctor proceeded to explain, the availability of donor hearts is not the most difficult challenge facing me, nor is it the most pressing reason for seeking out retransplant all the way across the country: it is my antibody profile that makes Cedars-Sinai an absolute imperative. The C1q antibody (along with many others I carry in my blood) would almost certainly run a rampant killing path within me, pummeling any donor heart that made its way into my chest and filling it with vasculopathy at lighting speed. It would not be fair to give me a precious new heart if the thing were fated to die soon after. I am one of the rare patients who need highly specialized antibody-destroying treatments to make heart transplant viable. And only Cedars-Sinai has the cutting-edge drugs and necessary expertise; Columbia simply doesn't.

Dr. Davis went on to assure me that transplant cardiologists from around the world refer their most challenging antibody patients to Cedars—specifically to the head of their program, Dr. Kobashigawa, who is *the* antibody expert in the country.

Even so, my heart may be too sick to hold on through whatever treatments this California doctor might administer. And with the particularly mighty antibody arsenal wrought by nearly twenty-six-years of a foreign heart, my case promised to be a daunting one, even to the Cedars team.

This is why Leja was so wrong about my getting a donor heart soon. I am compelled to remind her about the reality of my situation, this time using words from my new cardiologist at Cedars.

"I told you what Dr. Kobashigawa said the other day about my antibodies. Fourteen percent of the population—that's all I've got open to me right now," I say.

"He said antibody treatments will help to you. And remember, the doctor said to you about a patient with many antibodies—only *two* percent of the population can donate to him! But this person got a new heart!"

"Yeah, well, Dr. Kobashigawa is not telling me about the twenty other patients with really high antibodies who died last year because they couldn't get a matching heart in time."

Leja pulls her chin into her neck, and her lips begin to tremble. This is her cry pose.

I infuse my voice with tenderness now. "Look, Leja, I've learned never to take a doctor's *I have a patient who* tale at face value. You know I am not a person who will kid myself with stupid hope . . ."

"Hope is not stupid!" she snaps. "Hope is why I am here in America! You said no, it will not be that I am here, but it is happened!"

What had happened was a stroke of luck that allowed Leja to move to the United States with her daughter, Kima, and stay here forever— legally. This came about at first through sadness; Leja's brother fell ill and lost his job, which meant he could no longer provide housing and food for Kima, who attended a university in Croatia while Leja worked abroad. There was no turning to the girl's father for immediate help; he had left the country many years earlier. Her only option was to return home to Croatia, find work, and rent an apartment. But there were no jobs to be had, and before too long the money she'd saved started to run out. Desperate wishes and dreams whirled round in her head until they petered out and sank into hopelessness: if only she and Kima could come to the United States and become citizens. When I called every few weeks, she wept from the futility: "There is nothing what to do!"

Then one day, in her determined Leja way, she landed on something abruptly and went after it like a shot. "I will use it, my mind," she told me, and made a firm decision to stop all her useless dreaming and start up some powerful, directed visualization. She discovered a free website that allowed her to select specific affirmations that would run like a news ticker across her computer screen. Twice a day, she would sit for twenty minutes and focus on them, emptying her mind and inviting their messages into her unconscious, which she believed was connected to an unseen force of the universe. Or something.

I didn't really understand when she described it to me on the phone.

But the enthusiasm I heard in her voice was much better than the despondence that had taken hold for too many weeks.

"These are my affirmations," she told me, and read off her list: "'Good things are coming to me very soon. I will have a lot of money. I will move with my daughter to America and get a good job. I will be happy.'"

Upon hearing these, I knew what to do with my brand-new hardcover copy of *The Secret* that a friend had made the mistake of buying for me. There was no way I could bring myself to believe in the supreme power of positive thinking, which was the essence of the book. My body had defied optimism's efficacy too many times, like when I told my twenty-four-year-old self that the pounding palpitations I felt while walking up the spiral staircase from law school lobby to first-floor classroom would go away if I just sang to myself *"I am woman, hear me roar"* as I climbed. Ridiculous! After a week of singing and panting, I heard the words *heart failure* for the first time.

I mailed *The Secret* to Leja in Croatia. She was thrilled.

With a new how-to book in hand, Leja's affirmations soon graduated to physical form: handwritten Post-it notes and cutouts from magazines depicting her deepest wishes in full color. Leja started believing that if she devoted herself to giving silent blessings to people whom she might otherwise dislike, disregard, or feel sorry for, the good will she had put out into the universe would come back to her doubly strong. No matter the apparent lack of return on investment of time and energy, *The Secret* had a die-hard believer in Leja—at first.

"But I *will* come to America!" she told me two months later, through sobs. Her visualizations still had not become real life. Money was in shortest supply. All that *Secret* stuff had left her with nothing to hold onto but continued hope—and this made me almost regret giving her the book.

"Enough, Leja. I think it is time to look at your life just as it is and somehow make the best of it. You and your daughter will never go hungry—don't worry, you can count on Scott and me. Just please, stop wishing for something that will never come true."

She paused and blew her nose. "I *will* win the green card lottery! I will win it and come to America," she said, discounting the advice I had just given her. "Do you check the mailbox carefully?" She had applied for the US immigration lottery, whereby a tiny number of green cards are allotted to entrants from certain countries each year. The results would be sent to my home address.

"I get the mail every day, Leja. But forget about that, please. The odds of winning are ridiculous. You need to start accepting reality. Your life is and will always be in Croatia."

"No," she answered, "it will not be."

Three weeks later, there was an official government letter in my mailbox.

Leja had won.

"Don't worry about the details. Just come," I told her. "I'll find you an apartment and set it up—everything will be waiting for you when you get here." This was a dream that I could actually help make real for my friend Leja. Her winning might have been something of a miracle, but setting up her new life here required concrete thinking and productive effort. I was good at that. And my friends would be happy to chip in; the pure joy of being part of this incredible effort was infectious.

Two months later, Leja and Kima arrived from Croatia and I drove them to their new apartment in a small Connecticut town, where Kima could continue her studies at a state college nearby. I'd already paid two months' rent and connected the telephone, Wi-Fi, and electricity. I'd spent full days waiting for mattress delivery and for the Ikea assembly team to come set up whatever furniture Scott and I were not able to put together ourselves. The night before Leja's arrival, I made two beds with sheets and comforters purchased by Jill, hung the towels Deirdre paid for, put away silverware and dishes from Lauren, and put down an area rug from Jane. I plugged in a coffeemaker, toaster, and microwave—a group gift from all of us. When Leja walked into the apartment, everything she and her daughter could possibly need was in place—right down to dish towels and a carrot peeler. And the refrigerator was stocked.

Two weary Croatian women stood in stunned silence just inside the doorway of the spotless, bright, fully furnished rental apartment that seemed to have dropped magically from the sky.

"You did for *us*?"

"Of course," I said.

Six years later, it would be Leja using these same words, *Of course*, and I would be the one to stand in speechless surprise. Scott and I had asked her to come to California with us and be the one constant friend among the rotation of spreadsheet visitors. She answered without hesitation.

Committing to us for an unknown number of months meant quitting a nanny job she had been unhappy with for some time. "You make it easy for me to leave now," she said to me in my kitchen that day, telling the truth but also trying to lighten the weight of guilt she knew I felt in asking her to turn her life upside down this way.

And as for Kima, who'd grown to adulthood and was now married? "She will do," she commanded. Scott and I assured Leja that we would use our frequent-flyer miles to get her back to New York every couple of weeks.

"I want very much do this for you," she told me, meeting my eyes with intensity even as she retreated into cry pose. "For many years, I want to pay back for all you did when I come with my daughter to America. I worry—how I can thank you? I wait. I wait. And now I know why. This is what I must to do. I am so happy!"

Leja was going to help save my life.

IT IS BEDTIME and I am brushing my teeth in the Jack-and-Jill-style bathroom that connects the master bedroom with Leja's. I will sleep alone tonight because Scott had to fly New York for an important meeting and some solid work at the office for a few days. This is the first night I have been without him since arriving in California three weeks ago.

Leja knocks at the bathroom door from her side. "Okay. Good night," she announces.

I send a toothpaste-garbled good night back and spit into the sink.

"If you need me tonight, you wake me up." She means this as an order.

"Right," I say, and a flash memory of Joy offering up sleep company overtakes me with a wave of queasiness. Armed with lines from Shakespeare, Poe, and Wordsworth, I can be as self-reliant as if I were in my bed in New York. I will refuse Leja just as I did Joy. "See you in the morning."

I get into bed and adjust the three pillows that have held me in a sitting position every night since I arrived here. The room tilt that I felt lying down in bed at home has become even more pronounced in this bungalow. And now that my new heart transplant team here at Cedars-Sinai has made clear exactly how severely and rapidly my heart is declining into critical failure, I have allowed myself to finally stop muscling my mind through breathing rituals that do not stand a chance.

Your disease is galloping along . . .

These were the words used by Dr. Kobashigawa, my new transplant cardiologist at Cedars, to describe what he heard when pressing his stethoscope to my chest for the first time. It was a tense moment: a doctor who had never listened to my heart before was going to make his first pronouncement on its state of beating. Would he be curt and withholding like Dr. Davis, my brusque transplant cardiologist of twenty-six years at Columbia in New York, who had taken to grimacing and pivoting away from me after hearing the sure sound of my heart's dangerous decline? Dr. K, I learned quickly, has a different manner—a perfectly proportioned buoyancy in the midst of medical horror that I can't help but marvel at as clinical grace. Grabbing hold of each side of his white coat, he pulls them across his body one over the other, drops his chin, and smiles into the delivery of medical assessments and directives that are never sugarcoated, but instead softened by his beneficent nature.

This talented human being of a doctor was even able to add just the right touch of spin after listening for the first time to my terrible heart sounds, where the normal, crisp bum-*bums* were replaced by the alarmingly telltale ba-da-*bums*—his *galloping along* bringing to my mind the image of a clippity-clop horse to displace the gray-clogged artery tree that had stalled there since appearing on the angiogram monitor.

And not only had Dr. K been skillful in disclosing the sound he heard; he also had been right about the speed of the disease it characterized. I now am markedly worse than I was when the airport taxi dropped off Scott and me at the bungalow.

Under the covers now, I open my laptop and rest it on my outstretched legs. I will return to a half-watched episode of *Scandal*, the mind-numbing TV show that Joy made me promise I would download and give a chance.

I press start and settle in.

And then . . .

Whoa.

What was that?

Suddenly I feel—odd. Weighed down. Or is it more like . . . the icy driveway crawl again? Punctured and deflated.

I put the computer aside and become very still, trying to separate myself from the body sensations and, instead of reacting, just observe. This is not the breathlessness or palpitations that have become part of my everyday. This is not a side effect I have come to expect of my transplant medicines. This is new—or, rather, it *was* new. The feeling is less noticeable now; maybe it is even gone. But I know that whatever it was, I did not overreact to it; I do not scare easily.

"You're fine, Amy," I say aloud.

I pull the laptop back toward me, rewind what I missed, and start again. I watch the rest of the show and then lean over to turn off the light on my night table. And there it is again. That feeling of what I can only describe to myself as *wrong*. I reach for my cell phone and tap to light the icons.

Clock.

Stopwatch.

I am going to time my pulse.

I periodically check the speed of my pulse and the evenness of its rhythm all through the day, every day, and have been doing so secretly since a denervated heart took up residence in my chest: under the table at dinner, with hands behind my back at the gym, under the covers next to Scott in bed—fingers against wrist or side of neck. And I never feel cowardly or overreactive for doing it. My unruly transplant heartbeat always feels on the verge of emergency; counting beats allows me the illusion of control.

I begin the ten-second count.

One beat, two, three, four . . .

And it stops. My pulse has dropped off and I cannot find it anymore.

Huh?

I reset the stopwatch for another ten seconds and press the go-to spot on my neck this time—pointer finger against artery.

One, two, three . . .

And it is gone again.

What is going on?

I reach my right hand all the way across my body and push my fingertips into the side of my left rib cage—this is where my heart sits, where the decades-old transplant and subsequent open-heart valve surgeries deposited and redeposited it. Placing my hand here is always the surest way to find my pulse quickly.

One, two, three, four, five, six . . .

Okay, there it is, I've got it now.

The tally: ten beats in ten seconds. Multiply that by six, and I've got my one-minute pulse count.

Sixty?

My pulse can't be sixty. That would be almost cutting it in half.

My heart has never done this before; it is always too fast, never too slow. In twenty-six years, I have not seen my pulse go below ninety-five at any time.

I reach across my torso once again in search of that reliable sensation of heart against rib cage. But even this is not yielding continuous beats anymore. My pulse keeps fading and returning, slowing and . . .

Stopping?

My heart is spiraling down and stopping.

I should wake Leja.

She will be alarmed. Overwhelmed. Frantic to do something.

This will mean going to the emergency room.

Do I want to go to the emergency room?

Alone here in bed at midnight without anyone beside me to witness or influence my choosing, I am free to make a slow, private, determined decision and follow it through to ultimate consequence. There will not be any *Amy, you have to go to the ER! You can't just die here!*

I can just die here.

I can't rid myself of the fundamental question.

I sit with this thought for a minute: *Am I going to do this California transplant thing or not?* Because if I am, then I will have to call one of the nurses I met this week—Emily, who takes care of patients on the heart waiting list—and let her know I am headed to the ER. And if not— *Well . . . Scott has that letter for Casey . . .*

This slow, vanishing pulse is making everything a little blurry now, a little dreamlike. A languid calm settles heavily into my shoulders and arms. I am reflecting softly on the hummingbird in the garden today—a very good sign, Leja was sure of it. But how can it be that I received the bird's rosy prediction just this afternoon and now my heart has taken a sudden drastic turn for the worse?

An answer makes its way to me through the fog: *Because—remember, Amy—it is good to be worse.*

Experience has taught me this about heart transplant waiting lists:

The closer you are to death, the more likely you will get a donor heart. The sickest patients move to the top of the list and, if they are lucky, hover just this side of dying until a heart comes through for them.

The hummingbird was not telling me that I would soon get better, then; it was saying I was about to get much, much worse.

If there has ever been a time to move forward, it is now—before my hovering lands me squarely in death. Once I'm there, all choices will disappear forever.

I swing my legs off the bed and call out with whatever breath I can put behind it, "Leja, I need you!"

4

A very young-looking man in sneakers and a knit tie approaches my bedside saying, "I heard you had quite a night."

"Who're you?"

"Oh, sorry. I'm Dr. Baird, the resident here on Six South." He extends his hand.

"I don't shake. Immunosuppressed. And you're a giant germ in a white coat."

"I wouldn't doubt it, *heh-heh* . . ." He's looking down at the ground, chuckling, closing his eyes behind long dark lashes.

Too adorable. That's what I'm thinking. This guy is what Jill and I would've called cute thirty years ago. He lifts his face into a wide white smile, glowing like a high school valedictorian—or a middle school one. There's no hint of his needing to shave that chin anytime soon, which doesn't stoke my confidence.

"Is Dr. Kobashigawa coming to see me?"

"He's making rounds this morning. Should be here within the hour."

"I'll do the intake with him then, thanks."

"I'd like to examine you real quick first, if that's okay."

"It isn't."

Ahem, ahem.

Jody clears her throat and shifts in her chair beside my bed—right ankle over left knee, and switch—reminding me that I've got an audience. "Okay, okay, sorry," I say, sweeping my hands from side to side, shooing away my own words, resetting. "I'm not at my best right now. This is scary and freakin' awful, you know, Doctor, um . . ." I lean forward to look at the laminated ID tag hanging from his neck. "Baird, right, Dr. Baird. I was admitted through the ER after midnight. My heart keeps slowing down."

He gestures toward a folded sheet of paper sticking out of his coat pocket. "Yes. It's here on the overnight monitoring report." I'd been hooked up to a telemetry monitor—a constant EKG watched carefully by a central station on the cardiac floor. "Your heart is . . . well, it's failing."

"Yeah, news flash, right?" I look over at Jody for corroboration on my mild sarcasm. She's got her chin to her chest, staring into her lap.

"I'd really like to examine you before I—"

"Wait a sec. I think it might be happening right now. I'm feeling . . . floppy. Light-headed, ugh, hard to breathe . . ." I launch into habitual self-preservation mode where I become an excellent teller of symptoms in an emergency situation so a doctor can more easily identify what's going on in my body and, with some luck, save me from it. All eyes shift to the monitor screen beside my bed—a jagged stream of heartbeat lines in green and orange moving left to right beneath a large blue number that shows my pulse rate. The number is going down, sliding in free fall like a stone through black water, no sign of where the bottom may be: *91 . . . 83 . . . 76 . . . 65 . . . 58 . . . 49 . . .*

"I don't feel so good . . ." My hand lands on my forehead—I'm sweating.

Jody jumps to her feet, arms crossed in front of her chest. I turn my head toward her, and our eyes meet in trepidation. "Do you, uh . . . think you should maybe go get someone?" she asks the young doctor.

"Let's just watch and wait a minute."

Two nurses rush in, without our summoning. "Oh, you're in here. Good," one says to him. Central station had alerted them.

"Just giving it a few."

I turn on my right side and gaze up at the monitor: *41 . . . 49 . . . 60 . . . 73 . . . 82 . . .* "Here it comes now," I say, and lie back down in bed. "I'm all right." Jody remains standing, shifting nervously foot to foot. The nurses leave.

"Yup, looks like you're back at ninety or so, which is . . . fine, " the doctor says, back-stepping toward the door. "Maybe I'll come later and take a listen to your heart after you've seen Dr. Kobashigawa."

I say okay, and he turns to leave.

"Excuse me, excuse me, Doctor, please," Jody calls out. "That can't just keep happening to her, can it? Should I get the nurse if her pulse falls again?"

"Amy's on telemetry. The station will call the floor and send someone right away if there's trouble."

"Oh, okay, oh, good. Thank you, Doctor. Thank you *so, so* much," Jody says, all earnestness and direct eye contact.

Her solicitousness makes me uncomfortable—even though I know to expect it. Jody is always so darn kind. So careful and deliberate in what she says. And while I am just now discovering the etiquette she brings to a hospital setting, this isn't the first time I've wondered at her steadfast considerateness and decorum: I've been with Jody amid a group of women on several occasions where a gossipy comment pulls everyone in—except her.

Did you get a load of Renee's dress at the party last night—could it have been any farther up her crotch?

Great body, but come on, we're not teenagers . . .

Even my teenager wouldn't dress like that.

Well, Brett sure couldn't keep his eyes off . . .
Andy too, and I gave him a kick.
Ha-ha-ha . . .

And then there was Jody: "Totally short, yeah, and not my taste at all. But Renee seemed to be having a fabulous time, and I'm all for happiness." A few words from Jody can dry up the juiciest chatter—just like that. I've never once heard a mean syllable slip from her lips.

But then, I haven't spent all that much time with Jody. She and her husband, Jack, live in Los Angeles and are friends of friends, really, and this connection has brought us together mostly for celebratory group gatherings and outings over the last ten years. We've hugged each other in good cheer, the way occasional friends do—*So good to see you!*—and clinked glasses around a decade of happy-birthday dinner tables. But we've never had a girls' lunch just us two, and I've never once called her to say, *I'm so sick today, I could cry.* Jody is a situational friend, not a close one, and the situations have all been fun.

But now the circumstances are the opposite of fun, and I feel a burden to hold onto Jody's high regard and show that even under great stress, I still exhibit qualities worthy of her and the girlfriends we share in common. Pressure to perform bears down on me now, just as it has in the past—a familiar tension between my strong drive to put on a good face and my desire to give myself a break while in the grip of critical illness. While I used to see this as a choice between kindness to others and kindness to myself, experience has shown me that the two are actually blended: by eking out grace in the toughest moments, I reap benefits in the form of a favorable opinion from the people around me. I must keep this reciprocity in mind while in the company of Jody, who has never seen me under the strain of medical emergency.

Alone together for the first time ever, our essential selves are no longer diluted by the group around us; suddenly we are individuals writ large and on display. Jody is already demonstrating that her fine character remains intact, even with my pulse dropping before her eyes; intense apprehension does not fray her lovely manners—*Thank you so much, Doctor, thank you!* But I, on the other hand, am on edge. I was propelled through the door of the Cedars-Sinai emergency room just hours ago, superwoman Leja gripping my underarm. My desire to sustain my best self is challenged by my fading heart, and weakened by the anxiety of being far from home and far from Scott. Frightful thoughts and memories have been drawn fresh to the surface after last night's experience, but Jody is not aware of all that has come before this, all that is flooding me now.

"I thought to myself last night on the way to the ER, *I might never see Scott again*," I start in, by way of explanation. Her eyes pop. Legs cross and uncross. "I almost died in an ER with Scott twenty-five years ago."

Jody pauses before answering, "I did not know that."

"Yeah, makes this slow-pulse thing look like nothing because back then, before my first transplant, my heart would totally flip out. I mean completely go racing and skipping, and they'd have to defibrillate me. Shock to the chest, *bang!* And you know what was really strange—no one asked Scott to leave the room when it happened. He stood at the far end of my stretcher and held my toes while they shocked the hell out of me."

Again, there's a long pause.

"That's . . . awful," she says. And I know she's got to mean it because, well, it's Jody, and she's kind to the core. But there's a blankness in her tone that irritates the hell out of me. How can delivery of the word *awful* be so damn deadpan? Is it because of her perfect politeness? Maybe she's making a point of not latching onto my defibrillation saga so I won't feel awkward in the wake of blurting it out.

Does she think I'm oversharing?

But she's got so many blanks that need filling in.

Everything I say and do in front of Jody in this hospital room is going to look pretty bad to her if I don't hurry up and open a few windows into my past. I'm worried that, without context, she might rethink her basic impression of me as an affable woman and not be willing to take our friendship to a higher, more real level. Jody is not like our New York friends who've become inured to my medical dramas and have figured out their role to play in them; Jody is just now getting her first glimpse at closest range. I'd hoped that Scott and I might be able to prime her and Jack a little bit when we had dinner at their house a few days after arriving in LA, but the evening passed without either of them asking a single question about my upcoming appointments at Cedars and what my place on the heart transplant waiting list might entail. When Scott and I pulled away in our rental car, I tossed up my hands. "What's with that?" I asked, and he said Jody and Jack probably didn't want to pry and were waiting for me to open up the conversation. But I had a different read on it: maybe they saw that I looked just fine on the outside and figured my condition couldn't be all that precarious—a reaction that frustrates me, but one that I have encountered enough times to shrug off.

I learned last night that I was wrong. Jody had raced from her house in Santa Monica to join Leja and me in the ER at midnight. Just thirty-five minutes after Leja's fretful phone call woke her from a deep sleep—"I need that you come here *now!*"—Jody burst into my curtained cubicle. "So sorry, so sorry! It took much longer than I thought!"

"No worries, it's great that you're here—and I mean *really* great . . ." I shifted my eyes toward Leja, who'd brought her hands up in prayer position and affixed her eyeballs to the heart monitor screen above my head. "Thank you for coming, Jo."

"Ames, I gotta tell ya, you are so welcome." Her kind eyes sparkled above the warm Jody smile that showed a full expanse of upper and lower teeth. I immediately felt the comfort and calm of her presence.

"And just so you know, Jack wanted to come, he really did, but—"

"No need for both of you to be here."

"Yeah, well, he took an Ambien at eleven."

"Oh."

"And so did I."

"Jody! A whole Ambien, and you're *here?*"

"Yup."

Leja leaned in. "What is this Ambien?"

"A sleeping pill," I said. "Jody, please tell me you took an Uber?"

"You know, Ames, I did not, and I will admit that to you right here at the Cedars-Sinai ER," she said, adding an undertone of humor to her guilelessness. "There was no way was I going to wait one minute for an Uber. I just jumped in my car."

"Nooo . . ."

"Yeah, but I'm good. I'm good!"

"You must be exhausted."

"Nah." She lifted her eyebrows and stared out like a doll. "I can push through it for a couple of hours. And then I'll Uber home, for sure."

"You do not look to me sleepy," Leja announced, bringing her nose to Jody's chin and inspecting upward. "Your eyes are very awake. You do the Botox, yes?"

"Leja, come on . . ." I said.

"I do not *do the Botox*, no," Jody answered, "but thank you for the compliment."

This was Jody's first introduction to Leja. I would have to fill in some blanks in this area as well, but not just yet.

It is a good thing, then, that Leja is not here with us this morning in these tense, tight quarters. She is driving to the airport to pick up Scott, who, within twenty-four hours of his arrival in New York, had to fly back. Last night was my first emergency room visit without him by my side, and I know he's sad and sorry for this. But I see it as a backhanded stroke of good luck, actually; I had no choice but to spare Scott this latest ordeal and its hauntings—and he will live lighter for it because, as we've both come to realize, heart emergencies never leave you. They stall and seep in, slip behind your mind's curtain and wait in the wings of your consciousness, always looking for an opportunity to jump onstage—when you glimpse the light blue sweater you happened to be wearing the day the ambulance whisked you to the hospital, or the nail polish color you had on when an ER nurse said, "Get that off, honey. We need to see if oxygen's circulating to your fingertips." So you push that sweater far back in your closet, and you toss that bottle of nail polish and swear off all other pale pinks that may cue the fright-ful flash of memory. But the more skeletons you've got vying for your attention, the louder they rattle. And the more near-death emergencies you accumulate, the less power you have against them.

And so it was in the ER at Cedars-Sinai last night with those de-fibrillator pads on either side of my spine. "Just in case!" the nurse said, summoning the ghost of ER defibrillations past, when twenty-five-year-old Scott stood beside the stretcher of twenty-four-year-old me while I asked to be spared and told Scott I loved him, in between jolts of electricity to my chest.

This time, I had to brave it alone. Well, not exactly alone—Leja and Jody were there too. And now that I've filled Jody in on my defibrillation history, I've also connected a jolt of meaning to the blue-and-white pads she glimpsed through the slit in my hospital gown last night. Perhaps this explains the reason for the lack of expression in her *That's awful* response: Jody was so horrified, she didn't know what to say. Perhaps once she realized the pads on my back were a symbol of dread, she lost her words. After all, the defibrillator ghost makes its icy pass through bystanders too.

We sit in silence now, our eyes checking the big blue number every few seconds.

"Dr. Lunchbox," I say, making an effort to cut through the tension.

"What?"

"The doctor who was just here. Baird. He's, like, eleven years old. I'm going to call him Dr. Lunchbox."

She laughs. "Oh my gosh, that's perfect! *So* young-looking! But nice, right? The guy seems really nice."

"I'm not going to call it to his face. Don't worry."

"Well, that is smart," she says, playfully.

I explain that Dr. Lunchbox is a resident, one of the young doctors on the hospital floor—maybe two or three years out of medical school—who act as liaisons to the attending physicians. "So in a complicated case like mine, Dr. Lunchbox isn't going to be making any important decisions. That's why he stood there just now and watched my pulse drop: he doesn't have the authority or the experience to come up with a plan to fix it. Dr. Kobashigawa will do that, and Lunchbox will learn."

She nods, and then nods again. "Uh-huh, I see . . ."

"You think I wasn't nice enough to him."

"No, I'd say you were . . . fine."

"Look. If Dr. Lunchbox listens to my heart, he'll be lost. No way he's ever heard a near twenty-six-year post-transplant heartbeat before. He'd be putting on a show for me—*Okay, stethoscope to chest now*—lots of acting—*Hmmm, yes, well*. And I'd have to help him along: *My cardiologist in New York says there's a split first sound, but Dr. K hears it as a ventricular gallop. And there's a murmur because my tricuspid's leaking again, but don't confuse it with a mitral valve rub, even though I've got a moderate to severe one of those going on too these days . . .*"

She opens her mouth in amazement. "You sound like a doctor!"

"Yeah. Well, believe me, I'm not happy about it. Drives me crazy when I know more about nuances in my heart sounds than the guy listening to them, and then I have to go through the motions and pretend I value his dumb-ass input. And he's the one who's supposed to take care of me if everything goes haywire! I tell you, it's scary shit to be me in the hospital."

She leans toward the bed and puts her hand on my arm, and I feel the heat of embarrassment rush to my cheeks. The casual, surface-type relationship I share with Jody has no pretext for letting honesty fly—especially when accented with curse words. I rush to redeem myself: "Sorry, Jody. I'm all hyped up, you know? In save-my-life mode . . ."

My cell phone rings. Scott and Leja have just pulled into the hospital parking lot. I tell Jody they'll be up here in less than five, and then rise slowly from the bed to retrieve a clean pair of black yoga pants from the closet.

Having made a rule against hospital gowns long ago, I've still got on the jeans and shirt I wore to the ER last night. A sick person dressed as a sick person becomes an even sicker person is how I've come to figure it. I've also noticed the medical staff perk up at the sight of street clothes on a bedridden hospital patient: even the busiest doctor can't help but pay a little more attention when encountering the apparent display of a staunch will to normalcy and wellness. This is why I asked Leja to drop off a pair of black leggings and a few tops before heading to the airport this morning. "Do I look really sick?" I ask Jody as I head to the bathroom. "I don't want Scott to think I've gone terribly downhill over the last twenty-four hours—he'll feel bad for going back to New York."

"No worries there, Ames. You don't even look like you should be here."

"Thanks, Jo," I call out, turning on the water so I can wash any tearstains from my face.

"Jodela!" He has arrived.

"Scotty!"

I hear the squeak of chair legs against linoleum tile. Jody is up and moving toward Scott. I step out of the bathroom and find them in an elongated hug. Leja stands off to the side, glaring with suspicion.

"Hi, love," I say, coming up behind him.

He turns and throws his arms around me. "Sweetie, I'm so sorry I wasn't here. How are you doing this morning? Did I miss Dr. K?"

"No, he'll be here in a few minutes. Sit beside me," I say, climbing on the bed and leaving half the length of it for him. We fall back against the propped pillows and immediately into our natural fit with my head tucked under his chin. This is my safe place, my greatest comfort. Scott's body—the health of it, the dependability—is an instant refuge and the source from which I have drawn strength again and again in the past. His nearness feels like hope.

I start to cry.

"I know this is hard for you," Scott says, "but let's wait for Dr. K." He runs his hand along my cheek.

"We can step out . . ." Jody says, turning toward the door. Leja doesn't budge.

"No, no. I'm just so relieved that Scott's here," I reply. He hugs me closer for a few quiet seconds before turning back to our guests.

"So, Jodela," he says, "what's new? How's Jackie?"

"I'm happy to tell you that Jack has a breakfast meeting nearby and should be here pretty soon, I think."

"We're going to need more chairs," I say. "Dad's coming." My seventy-nine-year-old father flew in from New York this morning as well and is likely on his way to the hospital by now. He'd volunteered to come to LA (without my mom, for now, due to her paralyzing fear of flying) and help out at the bungalow while Scott was away. "And Rabbi Borski's stopping by too."

"A *rabbi?*" Jody is surprised. She knows that neither Scott nor I have ever taken part in organized religion, let alone become active members in a Reform Jewish synagogue like she and Jack have. I explain that I reached out to the local Chabad—an Orthodox Hasidic movement.

"Chabad!" Jody gasps with disbelief.

"Strange, I know, but I talked a few times with a Chabad guy years ago. He was my friend's rabbi, and I gotta say, he made sense to me. He said something about my life and my suffering having a larger meaning that I can't see—like maybe I'm here on this earth to remind everyone to be darn grateful they're not me."

"Thanks a lot," Scott says.

"Except for you, honey. Everyone would want to be me so they could be with you." I mean this.

"Well, just be careful," Jody says. "My friend had a bad experience with a Chabad rabbi. He went wacky on her, wanted money, and got heavy-handed with the proselytizing. It was a little creepy."

I turn in surprise to my kindly friend. "Wow, Jody," I say with a smile.

"Hold it, I take that back. Chabad can't all be the same, right? Your rabbi could be totally different. He's coming here to visit you and that sure shows a lot of—"

In walks Dr. Kobashigawa. "Morning, morning!"

Scott rises from the bed, and I sit up and away from the pillows. Jody gathers her bag, signals to Leja with her chin, *Let's go*, and they slip out.

TWENTY MINUTES LATER, Jack and Jody crack open the door and peek around it. "Okay if we come in?" They've been waiting outside for Dr. Kobashigawa to leave.

Scott motions for them to join us.

Jack walks directly to my bed and sits beside my hip. "Hi, Ames," he says with a frown, taking my hand in his.

I'm crying.

"Can I get you something? How about some Carvel? I'll run out right now if you want." Jack and I share a love for soft-serve vanilla.

I laugh, snorting a little through my tears. "You silly, it's not even eleven." Jack grabs a tissue and dabs the corners of my eyes, while Scott and Jody talk quietly, forehead to forehead, in the corner.

Leja would not like the looks of this.

And she would not be entirely off base: there is a crossover of admiration between couples, to be sure, and it has been a constant over the years we've been friends. But it doesn't rise to attraction—not sexual attraction anyway. It's more like favoritism or harboring a soft spot for the spouse of a friend, and Scott and I happen to have it—each of us, respectively—for Jody and Jack. Almost every time we see them, Scott tells me, "I just love that Jody." It's her sheer good-naturedness, he says, and how she's so straightforward and charming at the same time. "Jody's a lot of fun, she's casual and comfortable, not all dressed up and made up, and I don't know why, but she makes me smile 'til my face hurts."

"Maybe it's because your smile is a lot like hers," I've told him, "spreads across your whole face." He seems to like it when I say that. I think Scott senses the natural fit between himself and Jody, with their deep-set eyes and brown-black hair, and the easygoing slump of their shoulders that makes them both so approachable. Everyone likes Jody the instant they meet her, and the same can be said of Scott.

"If I got swallowed by a whale and you had to pick one woman from our friend group, who would it be?" I asked him once, after a few days at the beach with Jody, Jack, and friends.

He answered immediately, "Jody. And you?"

"Jack."

"I thought so."

Scott and I would never know if they felt the same way about us, but it didn't much matter. There was nothing to act on, nothing to do. Just a little sparkle to enjoy every now and then. Just a little special appreciation, and the pleasure of being appreciated specially in return.

Jack brings my hand to his lips now and kisses it. "Wanna tell me what the doctor said?"

"He says I need to have a pacemaker put in. Today. To stop my pulse from dropping. They're going to fit me in as an emergency, maybe in an hour."

"The doctor says she's much worse. They're going to keep her in the hospital until a donor heart comes through," Scott says. "No more bungalow for Amy."

"This is actually a good thing—getting sicker. It moves me higher on the waiting list. But I don't want that friggin' pacemaker in my chest. It's crazy enough to live with someone else's heart pumping inside me, and now it's going to be controlled by a *battery*? I might as well be a robot."

Jody and Jack think I'm being funny, but I couldn't be more serious. Dread of needing a pacemaker has been a constant throughout my years with a racing, unruly transplanted heart. I even warned my Columbia cardiologist long ago, "Don't you dare even suggest a pacemaker—'cause I'd give it an absolute N-O." For me, the feeling is visceral and, I suspect, unusual among cardiac patients. I just can't help but feel that there's something alarming and even sickening about wedging a control device into a heart that's already been cut from one body and moved to another.

But the full intensity of my reaction is not to be shared with Jody and

Jack, not now. Boundaries may be moving fast in this hospital room, but in this moment my instinct is to pull back instead of try to explain myself. I have opened up to them more than enough already.

"Amy's not too happy about getting a pacemaker," Scott says.

"I don't have a choice. Dr. Kobashigawa said he's worried about cardiogenic shock."

Jody and Jack freeze in place.

Jody raises her hands by her ears, as if in a stickup. "Okay, Ames, I have absolutely no idea what that is."

"You don't want to know," Scott says.

"Death," I say.

Scott shoots me a look. "That's not likely to happen. Amy's getting a pacemaker."

Jody and Jack mumble how great that is, and thank God for pacemakers.

Just then my father appears in the doorway with Leja in tow. "Table for two!" he calls out.

Rabbi Borski shows up just behind them, crowding the space by the door. "Make it three!" he adds. There's no long coat, I notice. No tall hat either. Not even a stereotypical Orthodox beard. Instead, this rabbi wears a dark blue suit and matching tie. His salt-and-pepper beard is kempt and not very religious-looking. His expression is humble and friendly.

I hug my father, do the introductions around the room, and gesture for him and the rabbi to take a seat. Scott and Leja find spots to sit at the end of my bed. Jack and Jody lean against the wall. And as if the tiny hospital room weren't packed enough already, here comes Dr. Lunchbox.

"They're going to take you to the cath lab for your procedure in about forty-five minutes, all right?"

I nod and turn to my father. "I'm getting a pacemaker."

Leja jumps. "What is happened!" Scott gets up and whispers something to her that prompts instant composure, then walks over to my father and leans in for a few private words.

The room falls silent.

"Mets or Yankees?" It's Rabbi Borski. His voice crackles with light. "I take it you're all New Yorkers. Tell me, who's your team?

"Mets."

"Mets."

"Dodgers—the Brooklyn Dodgers, that is," my father says.

"Ah, you're from Brooklyn. Me too," the rabbi tells him.

"I grew up on President Street."

"President Street! What number?"

"Fourteen sixty."

The rabbi smiles. "My first cousin Abraham lives in that building."

My father's eyes cloud with nostalgia. He shakes his head. "Well, how about that. Talk about coincidence! I haven't seen the place in sixty-five years . . ."

"I'm sure my cousin would be happy to give you a tour sometime!"

"Ah, now there's a joke about that . . ." my father says, grabbing the opportunity to dig into his trove of Jewish humor. "May I share it with you, Rabbi?"

"Please do, yes."

"So Morris is alone on a desert island for a long time. He builds a house. A library for himself. And, *tzadik* man that he is, he builds not just one synagogue, but two beautiful structures to God. One day a sea-wrecked sailor washes up on the island, and—"

"'I wouldn't be caught *dead* in that synagogue!'" The rabbi finishes my father's joke.

There's laughter and knee slapping. Everyone is swept up in the fun of a stolen punch line.

"So you've heard that one before, Rabbi?"

"Heard it? I delivered it to my congregation at Rosh Hashanah service this year!" He pauses, looks to the ceiling, and thinks for a few seconds. "Okay, let me tell you about *this* . . . There's a church with a rodent problem, such a terrible thing, you shouldn't know from it. You familiar with this church?"

"I don't think so. Go on, Rabbi."

I scan the room: there's merriment, everyone encouraging the banter. But minute by minute, the scene is turning gruesome in my eyes: the toothy smiles all around, the popping eyes and reddened faces, the twisted sound of incongruous enjoyment. I zoom from face to face.

Don't you see me checking my pulse rate every few seconds?

Jody's eyes were no longer glued to the monitor along with mine: Is it that easy for others to be distracted from what's really going on in this hospital room?

I'm about to get a pacemaker put into my dying transplanted heart, for fuck's sake.

"Well, this church, it's right across the street from a synagogue that also has rats, you see. The priest and the rabbi use the same pellets to get rid of these creatures, but they keep returning only to the church. So one day the priest sees the rabbi and says, 'Do you still have rats in your synagogue?' and the rabbi tells him no, they're gone. 'Can I ask you then, Rabbi, how do you get them to stay away?' and the rabbi says, 'I bar mitzvah them and they never come back!'"

Laugher and more laughter. The room is positively jolly.

I manage a smile, but that's as much as I can muster.

"Why they do not come back?" Leja asks aloud.

No one seems to notice my loud exhale.

"Because after a kid is bar mitzvahed, he never goes back to temple again," Jody explains. "That's a great one, Rabbi!" She's beaming at him.

My father starts in immediately, "So Sadie comes home from shopping one day and finds her husband, Sam, in a chicken suit . . ."

"'Not on the Sabbath, Sam!'"

Another jump to the punch line.

I roll my eyes—but everyone is chuckling too heartily to notice.

My father and the rabbi continue on like this for some time, delighting the room. Finally, a nurse comes in to say, "I see you're very popular. Some crowd in here! Amy, dear, I've got a gown for you." She steps toward me and the chatter starts up again at a lower decibel. "You're going to have to put this on for your procedure. Open to the back, please."

I take the gown and rest it beside me. "Scotty, could you, uh . . ."

He understands.

"Hey, everyone, Amy needs to change . . ."

There's talk of heading for a quick coffee downstairs as they file out one by one.

See you later, Amy . . .

In a bit, Ames . . .

Be right back, hon . . .

Can I get you anything?

"No."

I sit quietly for a couple of minutes with no intention of replacing my button-down flannel shirt with the gray-blue gown just yet.

"Ames? Okay if I come in?" It's Jack.

"Of course."

He steps into the room and shrugs. "I didn't go with them. Wanna take a quick walk with me in the hall?"

"Okay." I leave the gown on the bed and slip the loop of my telemetry monitor over my shoulder like a purse. I'm leery to leave the room, but I can be a little bit brave knowing that the monitor will still be picking up every heartbeat. "Let's go," I say. There's a box of yellow surgical masks mounted by the door frame. I reach for one and secure it behind my ears. "Got to wear this. Hospital germs out there." We make a right turn and step into the wide white hallway.

Jack takes my hand.

"I need to go at grandma pace, sorry."

"No problem, Ames. I'm just happy to be with you."

The corners of my mouth turn up beneath the germ mask. How can I not smile at Jack's sweetness? He let the others go for coffee without him just so we could have a walk together. We're not going to talk about pacemakers. We're not going to speculate about how long I might have to wait for a heart now that I've been hospitalized indefinitely. There won't be any forced joke telling. Jack and I don't have to speak at all; it's plenty nice just carrying a feeling between us.

It's special.

"I gotta stop, sorry." It's been only about twenty feet. We drop hands in front of a large window looking out over an expanse of Los Angeles. I try to catch my breath.

Jack becomes an instant tour guide, pointing here and there. "That's Century City, and if you go straight down you'll get to Santa Monica . . ." After a few minutes, I tell him I'm good to walk again and we head back to the room. Stepping inside the door, we see everyone is back in place, just as they'd been earlier.

Leja is glaring at Jack.

My father offers me his chair, saying, "Maybe you'd like to stay out of bed," and I take a seat beside the rabbi. Within seconds, a young man in a Cedars-Sinai uniform comes in.

"I've got a stretcher outside to go to the cath lab." He pans the room. "Uh . . . who's the patient?" Since I'm still dressed in leggings and a plaid shirt, there's no way to tell I'm the sick one.

Ha-ha-ha-ha . . .

I don't join in the laughter.

"It's me," I say.

"I'll be in the hall when you're ready to go. Family and friends, you can wait in the waiting area while she's in the cath lab."

There's movement around the room, everyone gathering their things.

Rabbi Borski rises to his feet. "I'd like just three minutes alone with Amy, if that's all right."

My father answers for the group, "Sure. See you in the hallway, honey."

Seconds later, they're all gone.

The heavy door thumps closed.

"Well then," the rabbi says, and pulls out a black leather-bound book from his briefcase. "A prayer."

I'M ON MY back, gliding beneath a track of fluorescent lights. A cath lab nurse is wheeling my stretcher through an interior hallway that leads from the holding area to the procedure room, and I haven't got a new poem.

There wasn't time to memorize one and there's no comfort in harking back to a recent recitation that brought me no good luck. I'm going to have to scrape the bottom of the mind game barrel—fast.

All right—how 'bout let's play "What's different here?" This is my first time in a cath lab that's not Columbia's, after all; what's different here at Cedars? Not my best invention, but it will have to do. Carefully narrowed focus is the only trick I've got right now.

Okay, so . . .

Lining the hallway, there's a stretch of horizontal hooks where X-ray protective clothing hangs at the ready. Some items have designs: purple swirls, camouflage, tiny dots in happy colors (*These belong to the nurses,* I'm thinking, *they like to doll up their gear at Columbia too*). Then comes the lineup of scrub sinks—deep stainless steel basins with foot-pedal controls and large hanging vats that dispense some kind of skull-and-bones hospital-grade soap with the touch of a forearm. Two doctors stand side by side chatting, their hands covered in bubbly froth.

What are the sinks doing in the hallway? At Columbia, they're inside each procedure room.

My stretcher comes to a stop, and I'm watching the doctors rinse and re-bubble, scrub-brush their nails—rub, rub, rub—and rinse again, this time with fingers pointed down (*so the germs slide away from the body and down the drain—Columbia doctors do this too*).

I should remember to do a final downward rinse at the end of my hand washing . . .

The nurse hits a silver square on the wall. A pair of double doors opens to the cath lab, and she pushes me inside. It's freezing in here.

Two large flat-screen monitors. Dozens of meter-length catheters in sterile wrap hanging inside glass-front cabinets. Steel cart with surgical implements lined up. *Yup, just the same as Columbia.*

The narrow procedure table is set in the center of the room.

"Can you slide yourself over, or do you need help?" the nurse asks.

"Done it a hundred times. Literally. I'm great at the stretcher-to-table switch," I tell her, pushing up with my hands and shifting my body from one long cushioned surface to the other. But this time the simple motion sucks all the oxygen out of my lungs. This has never happened to me before.

I'm so much sicker now than I ever was at Columbia.

Mind game over.

"Give me a minute before I lie down?" I say to the nurse, hoping it will be enough time to regain my breath. She nods and turns to greet the doctor who's just come in—a small, quick-moving man with wiry gray hair.

"I am Dr. Wayne. Hello, Mrs. Silverstein."

"You can call me by my first name if you like. I'm Amy."

"Hello, Mimi."

"No, it's *Amy*," I say, and then immediately think to correct myself for fear that he might call me "Itsamy." Dr. Wayne's speech is choppy, perhaps due to his jittery manner.

"Today I will put in a pacemaker."

"Yeah, I guess that's what you gotta do."

"I'll give you medicine for sleep . . ."

"I'm not going to sleep."

"Not really sleep. Just very, very relaxed. *Like* sleep."

"Nope. No sedation at all. I do everything without sedation unless it's a surgery. This isn't a surgery, is it?"

"Not exactly surgery, but—"

"Good then. No sedation."

The doctor whirls away from the exam table and mumbles under his breath loud enough for the nurse and me to hear: "No sedation! For a pacemaker! Sheesh . . ." He heads into the hallway to scrub up. The nurse remains behind, tending to an array of syringes and small metal utensils.

"I don't want to give anyone a hard time," I tell her, "but I've had lots of experience staying awake through hard stuff. And I don't like being put out."

"You wouldn't really be *out*. Just relaxed. We'd be giving you some Versed . . ."

Versed! No way.

I'd like to ask her how many times she's had Versed, because I've had it plenty and it's a nasty sedative.

Instead, I press my lips closed. *Check your attitude, Amy.*

That's what Scott told me just before we headed out to LA. We had a long talk one evening, mulling the challenges we knew would be coming and trying to anticipate what else we might face. "If you're going to die," Scott said, "and let's be honest, you might—you need to think about how you want to act at Cedars, how you want to hold yourself in the end. With your friends—do you want to be loving, or bitter and angry? And with the doctors and nurses—do you want to earn their respect for the way you've lived these twenty-five transplant years, or do you want to show how you've been wrecked by them? It's all about how you want to be remembered," he said.

This was not the first time that Scott had attempted to remind me of my better nature. There had been plenty of instances through the years when frustration and fear overtook me, transforming qualities like self-advocacy, determination, and attention to detail into alienating misbehaviors. The constancy and complexity of transplant-related illnesses would crescendo from time to time, to a point where it felt unbearable—and where it would imbue me with a distorted sense of self-righteousness: *Give me a break—I can't be bothered with decorum. I'm too sick.* And then I would rage against Dr. Davis's missteps, calling him *inane*, or I wouldn't pick up the phone for days when friends called to check in, or I'd yell at Scott for no reason at all and then cry and cry

and cry. Then came the heavy regret: "Scotty, I'm just so, so sorry . . ."
and he would close his eyes and shake his head. "You're dealing with
unbelievably scary stuff, I know. But you've got to find a way to stop tak-
ing it out on the people around you." If I didn't, he said, I would send
everyone scurrying away.

I tried to do better. With each successive medical crisis, I got a
little more adept at keeping my fear from spiraling into anger and
spurring me to lash out. But I found that the success of my efforts
was only proportional to the health challenge at hand: the more life-
threatening it was, the less I was able to contain my angst. What de-
gree of self-control, then, would I manage to exert in the face of this
retransplant?

I was yet to find out. But it spooked me to notice that, in light of
what awaited us in California, Scott had rephrased his usual advice
about how I might carry myself in the hardest of circumstances. For
the first time ever, he was framing his words in a context of finality,
asking me not about how I might want to be perceived but rather
remembered.

I just want to be remembered without everyone misunderstanding me.

I know this doesn't speak to the self-reflection Scott hoped for. But
right now, this is what comes to mind as I contemplate how I might
explain to this nurse my aversion to Versed. I know my stance is un-
usual; when patients hear that they're getting a drug to help them relax
before an invasive procedure, they see no reason to object. But long,
hard-earned experience has taught me this: Versed messes with your
mind. It's a powerful, tricky sedative that makes you think you've slept
through the procedure when actually you were awake the whole time.
Versed is, simply, a forgetting drug, but its powers of erasure are im-
perfect. Somewhere in your mind (and certainly in your body) there is
a flicker of awareness that something happened to you (for instance,
you might have been screaming in pain throughout the procedure), but
you can't quite get at it, so an anxious ambiguity scratches at you and
festers. There is a cost to not being able to access and process our own

pain and suffering—some might call this post-traumatic stress. I've experienced it myself, and this is why I've come to insist on keeping things where I can see and process them—without Versed.

I share my thinking with the nurse.

She walks from the tray to my stretcher and lowers her voice. "I agree with you. And too much Versed isn't good for your brain cells either." She taps her head. "But Amy, I've never seen a patient do a pacemaker implantation without sedation. It's going to be rough."

"I hope you're wrong. But thank you."

Dr. Wayne stomps back in and comes to a stop by my left shoulder. "I'm going to have to give you a lot. Of lidocaine. Because you said *no sedation*. Sheesh."

"Fine with me." I don't mind multiple lidocaine shots. I've accumulated three or four hundred of them for localized numbing in all the biopsies and angiograms I've had. From experience, I know that if the doctor gives the first shot slowly—alternating a bit of needle with a bit of lidocaine—subsequent injections will become quickly pain free.

BANG!

Dr. Wayne slams the first shot into the left side of my collarbone.

"Ow!"

"That hurt you," he says.

"My gosh, yes. *Ow*. In New York, the doctor gives a little bit of lidocaine at a time so . . ."

"I said you would need a lot of shots. Because of no sedation."

BANG!

This one feels like it has vengeance behind it. I clench my teeth, determined not to give in.

BANG and *BANG*—two more in rapid succession.

That's it.

"Ow! Ow! Oh my God! I can't take it!" I'm weeping now, and I can't believe I'm crumbling this way. I don't cry from pain. What pierces my armor this time is the frightening vulnerability I feel at the gruff hands of a masked stranger in a cath lab far from the one I've known for twenty-six years. Reciting poetry couldn't possibly combat what is looming over my body at this moment. A nurse's tender glance would bring me no ease. The reassuring touch points I've come to rely on give way to stabs of surprise—each one of them another fiery agony. I have never known cath lab procedures to be scenes of horror, but I feel myself here in the grip of a ghoul.

"It's too much for you. Right?" Dr. Wayne glares.

"No, I'm strong as hell. I've been on a hundred cath lab tables. It's you! You've got terrible hands—has anyone ever told you that? You suck at this! Just give me the damn Versed." Oh, I've really let loose now. I sure don't want to be remembered like this, but I've lost all control.

"Oh, *now* you want it? I have to call anesthesia. It will take, I don't know, an hour. For them to get here. Because you said *no* sedation!"

I pause, taking a few seconds to muster a conversational tone. "You need an anesthesiologist to administer Versed? In my experience, the nurse just puts it in my IV—at least that's how they do it in New Y—"

"In New York! In New York!" He galumphs away from the exam table, waving his hands over his head. The nurse follows, and I'm alone.

I've never been left alone in a cath lab before.

Does this mean I'm on my own for the next hour? Isn't someone coming back?

No.

They've left me lying flat with the slightest pancake of a pillow under my head. Within a minute, I know, I'm not going to be able to breathe.

What will I do? I'm going to have to sit up to catch my breath.

But that will ruin the layers of sterile draping they've laid across my body so carefully; they'll be madder at me than they already are. I've got to stay put until the anesthesiologist arrives—one hour.

That's sixty minutes. Three thousand six hundred seconds . . .

I start counting.

One, two, three . . .

Soon my head feels fuzzy. My eyes close against my will. I lose count. I think my pulse must be dropping, but I can't place a fingertip on my wrist to check it because the nurse secured my arms tight against my sides before wrapping me in sheeting . . .

And I can't turn my head far enough to see the blue number on the monitor . . .

And I can't sit up . . .

And I can't breathe . . .

And I'm alone—in this room, in this terror, in a body that is speeding toward its end.

Serious illness reveals the infinite depth of solitude. I settled into its bottomlessness years ago, and yet the panic of isolation overtakes me still.

And there's Scott and Jody, Jack and my father and Leja—all of them sitting together in the waiting room right now without any idea that I'm barely holding on in here. How am I going to explain to them—that the doctor was rough, that he plunged needles into me like tranquilizer darts into a grizzly bear. That I lay flat on the exam table in need of an oxygen mask, but no one was there to help.

I could have died. No, really, listen to me—it was beyond what I could handle in there!

They won't feel the weight of it. They'll find a way to lighten whatever I say to them. *We bar mitzvah the rats and they never come back! Ha-ha-ha-ha!*

Stop that cackling! I can't stand the damn gaiety!

I've lost count again—*eighty-uh-two . . . eighty-nine?*

I'm confused. Woozy.

The double doors open and someone rushes in.

My eyelids flutter.

I feel my mouth fall open.

Within seconds, the green-clad people descend, ghoulish in their masks and puffy caps, gloves and X-ray shields. There are here to slice into my skin, slide their control wires into my heart. One of them pulls back the sheeting from my left shoulder, where scattered injection punctures still ooze blood onto my naked breast.

The Versed sweeps through my IV . . .

Where are my clothes?

What happened to my voice?

Why can't I remember?

I OPEN MY eyes to a familiar hospital room. Scott is the first to notice.

He sits on the bed and puts his hand to my cheek. "Hi, honey."

I stare past him, unfocused. Lingering Versed makes it easy for me not to respond.

"She's awake!" Leja shouts.

Shoes shuffle across the floor. I sense bodies gathering at the left side of my bed.

"Amy, honey. I'm right here."

Scott again.

I don't move my eyes. I don't speak.

He smooths my hair. "You're back in bed now. Everyone's with you. The procedure is all done."

All done? What happened to me in that room? . . . Will it ever be done?

Beneath vacant eyes, I'm trembling—terror is still coursing through me. But as I start to get my bearings, I realize that I'm also boiling mad.

"It's the anesthesia." My father's voice.

No, it isn't.

"Let me try." Jack takes Scott's place beside me on the bed. "Ames, it's Jack. Say something to me. Just say, *Hi, Jack.* I'd like that, Ames. Ames?" He looks up at Scott, "She's not right. Should we tell someone?"

Scott picks up my hand. "Limp," he says. "She's not responding at all." Panic begins to rise in his voice. "Let's get a doctor in here. Hey, Jody?"

"Yeah?" I hear her voice from over by the door. This silence I'm perpetuating, it's stirring everyone up in a punishing way. Terrifying them second by second. Causing pain and fear where there needn't be any. But I don't know if I'm actually capable of responding at this moment. I'm not even sure I'm alive. The separation I feel from my own body is so severe, so alarming—the thought crosses my mind: *Am I in shock?*

Whatever I'm in, it's an altered state, the likes of which I've never experienced; for the first time in my adult life, I've lost the desire to wrangle words and express myself. My mind is doing somersaults. Thoughts are tumbling like Ping-Pong balls in a bingo cage; each one bears a piece of vital information right there on the surface, but I can't possibly call it out. The whirl of clack-clacking has to stop—only then can I reach into the jumble, make sense of what I pull from it, and speak aloud to those who are asking to hear my voice.

"I'll find the resident," Jody says. I hear the door close behind her.

Jack tries again, louder this time, "Ames! Ames! Please, just one word."

"Squeeze my hand!" Scott calls out.

My mind goes soft again.

He lets go, and my arm collapses beside me.

"Doctor's on his way," Jody says. Her voice grabs my conscience. This isn't the good impression I wanted to make on her today, but I can't bring myself to respond. The lingering effects of Versed won't shake.

Soon there's a stethoscope against my chest. A penlight in my eyes. It's Dr. Lunchbox. He addresses the room: "I don't know what's going on with her exactly. I'll give Dr. Kobashigawa a call. He'll want to order a brain scan . . ."

I'm still working myself out of a stupor, finally gathering the effort to respond. "No scan," I manage to mumble.

"*Amy!*" Scott squeaks with emotion.

"Yeah, I'm here." Even I can hear the shrug in my voice—it's sort of like, *Okay, you got me.*

Scott's eyes narrow with incredulity. "Did you just . . ." He pauses with his mouth open. "Were you able to . . . but you didn't?"

I don't answer.

"Why would you do that? Didn't you see how worried we were? And you just kept pretending that you couldn't speak!"

"I wasn't pretending."

I was traumatized, I want to say. *I'm in shock.* But I don't.

The doctor slinks out. Jack steps back from the bed. I lift my gaze and focus for the first time on Jody, who's pacing back and forth in short strides over by the door, her arms folded tight against her chest. She pivots to face me and our eyes meet.

I wince.

What she must think of me now . . .

I had hoped Jody and I might have days and weeks to ease into a closer friendship, that my time in LA would mean we'd get to know each other on a deeper, more meaningful level. I worry that I've gone and set things back for us; Jody probably thinks I've acted cruelly to-day—or that I'm crazy.

But I lost my words, don't you see? I never lose my words . . .

What happened in the cath lab—it's not the same as the medical trauma that I've become used to over these transplant years, the kind you can tamp down or maneuver around pretty well, even though it sticks with you. No, this experience today—being disempowered in such a terrifying way—it doesn't just stick. It breaks you.

A pacemaker inside me. Versed in my veins.

Needle-stab splotches spreading black and blue across my chest.

Empty cath lab.

Gasping, gasping . . .

I can't find a way to wrestle these horrors to the ground. There's no stomping them out. My mind gives way to the spinning bingo cage again, little white balls encoded with memories of medical chaos—whirling, blurring. But this time, I can't bring myself to reach into the bin and grab hold of a few, name them and reframe them as I have in the past to control the terror they carry. In this moment, the thought of even the smallest effort for self-preservation is exhausting. I can't help but sink now; I've been paddling too hard and for too long.

The cost of survival is decimating me, right here, right now.

I turn my head away from Jody and find Leja on my right with her palms over her eyes, weeping. It was just one day ago that we laughed together in the garden, sharing what I'd learned about hummingbirds (my spirit animals, as she's since come to call them), whose portents we hoped would connect my fate with an unbounded energy—soaring, zooming, persevering. But what I didn't share with Leja were the words in the essay that drew the closest and truest parallel between these birds and me. These poor little birds would be beaten down and broken by their very existence:

> The price of their ambition is a life closer to death; they suffer more heart attacks and aneurysms and ruptures than any other living creature. It's expensive to fly. You burn out. You fry the machine. You melt the engine.
>
> BRIAN DOYLE, *"Joyas Volardores"*

He told me that God has a book. And in this book he keeps a list of people who are going to die soon.

I know almost nothing about Judaism, so I don't exactly buy it.

"What we need to do is get you off that list," he said.

"How?"

"Oh, but there is a way."

We would use my Hebrew name. Seems the secular name I carried with me into the hospital was on that bad list in God's book. But my Hebrew name, "Well, that, you see, is not."

I didn't have a Hebrew name to give him.

"So we will choose one now," Rabbi Borski said. "What name would you like?"

I told him I knew of a Chabad woman named Ahuva.

"Means 'loving.' That's very nice for you, yes, and let us add to it the name Leiba. Means 'heart.'" He pronounced the final T sound with such emphasis that I felt it sharp in my chest. "Ahuva Leiba—a loving hearT."

There it was again—that T.

The prayer was short; the rabbi recited lines in Hebrew and I repeated them back to him.

"That's it?"

"That's it."

We walked into the hallway together and I climbed onto the stretcher. As I rolled toward the cath lab, the echo of his voice followed me down the long hallway. "Good-bye for now, Ahuva Leiba. You will live long. You will get your hearT."

5

———

arlier this morning—before the doctors had come in, and be-
fore I'd heard them speak the words *cardiogenic shock* and
pacemaker—Jill composed a group email and sent it to me for
approval. The ultimate recipients would be the women who'd signed on
to the spreadsheet, and each of their visits would have to be moved up
by about two weeks due to last night's emergency and what appeared to
be a quickening downslide of my heart. As the first friend on the sched-
ule, Jill would scramble to get on an early-evening flight, throwing a
few things into a suitcase before leaving for work in hopes of amending
her existing ticket and heading straight to the airport at day's end.

"That's a huge change fee, I'm so sorry," I told her when she called
after speaking with the airline's customer service. "It might not be
worth the money for you to come right now."

"Forget the money. I'm coming," she told me, but I couldn't ignore
the additional dollars.

"Did you try to get that emergency-discount thing—airlines do that
sometimes."

"Tried. The rep said it has to be a family member. A friend's not

good enough, apparently. So I pushed back, you know, 'But, but, but—
she's my *best* friend . . .'"

   Best friend.

   I couldn't be sure whether this was one of Jill's tactical ploys to tug
a heartstring and wrench a fee waiver out of this customer service rep,
or whether she'd meant it in earnest. As close as Jill and I are, we've
never put that kind of comparative label on our friendship. In fact, it
has seemed to me that dodging the *best friend* designation has been
quietly intentional on both our parts—at least in our adult years when
we have found opportunities to show each other, casually but assur-
edly, that we're past labeling our relationship. And so now, reliably,
whenever Jill introduces me to someone, she says, "This is Amy . . .
my *oldest* friend," then compresses her voice into thin falsetto, "and
I'm talking *old*—what are you now, Amy, ninety-two? And doesn't she
look just super!" I play along, hunching my back: "Oh, I'm ancient all
right!"

   At fifty years old, we know there is nothing to be gained from rating
or categorizing friends for elucidation, and Jill and I are plenty secure
in our devotion to each other. And besides, just what is a *best* friend
anyway? Jill and I have a deep connection that stands apart from our
other friendships. This is evidenced in part by her role as my secretary
of communications (a.k.a. medical-information scribe, reporter, and
disseminator), which has been part of our relationship since my first
transplant. Whenever I emerge from a heart biopsy or angiogram, or
when I step out of a doctor's office after hearing hard news, I rely on
Jill to save me from having to gather myself and repeat the same story
five, eight, ten times to others. She is always eager to take over commu-
nications to the girls in particular, typing my words into an email as I
speak them, transforming occurrences into paragraphs of clear facts,
and circling back to ensure she's got it all correct before pressing send.
I don't know if this is the kind of thing that makes a friendship *best*, but
it sure does feel great to ease myself down into it—*ahhh*—like a warm
bath of trust and comfort.

Tonight she will write another one of these meticulous notes—this time from my hospital room, which will be a first for both of us. I don't usually talk to Jill until I've had time to digest some of the effects and burn off some of the anger and fear, and even then the buffer of a cell phone has always separated us. What Jill and I are about to embark on in this California hospital room, then, is a whole new kind of interaction: three days of togetherness, which means undiluted emotions and interactions, live and up close. I won't need to give her a highlight-reel recap; for once, Jill will be on the field right along with me, minute by minute, more able to assist in taking on my medical challenges than any friend before—perhaps sliding into position, then, as my true best.

The game begins now—10:15 p.m. Scott and my father just left to grab a very late supper together. Leja's text pushed them out the door moments ago; she's picked up Jill at the airport, and they're a quarter mile from the hospital. This leaves me only a few short minutes alone, my first since waking up from the pacemaker implantation some eight or nine hours ago. I close my eyes and smile inwardly: *Jill!*

A few minutes later, a sharp call from the doorway startles me: "We can come!" Leja means this as a question.

"Of course . . ."

Leja enters first, followed by Jill, who puts down her carry-on bag and freezes in place. I'm sitting up in bed, propped against pillows; all is clean and orderly. But Jill looks at once overwhelmed. Surprised. Frightened. She forces a smile, but I sense the intonation of a question in the way she speaks my name: "Ames?" I look different in this California hospital room than I did on my sofa back in New York.

I shrug my shoulders as if to say, *Sorry.* "Jilly. Hi."

Leja has an announcement: "I am tired. Three times today to airport. I will go now to bungalow."

"Sure, see you tomorrow," I say.

"You need clean underwear. I bring them in the morning."

"Thank you, Leja."

"I bring tea for you. Or hot chocolate? At nine thirty." She whips away the throw blanket from my legs, gives it a good shake, and then sets it down again with precision.

Jill is still standing a few feet from the bed—silent.

"Hot chocolate would be great. Thanks, Leja, good night." I turn my head to meet Jill's intense stare, which hasn't left me since she walked in. I raise my hands to my ears. *"What?"*

She steps toward my bed, and I see that her eyes are filled.

"Is it the bandage?" A four-by-four-inch gauze pad secured with clear medical adhesive peeks out from my pajama top, just beneath the front of my left shoulder. "It's not bleeding through, is it?"

"No, no, it's not the bandage." She sits on the edge of the mattress, still managing to keep from spilling tears. "It's just . . . you look . . ."

"Bad, huh? I put on a little mascara early this morning, but I haven't checked the mirror since then. I got a pacemaker, that's what the bandage is for . . ."

"I know. I spoke to Scotty."

"So you heard he's really upset with me because I, ah . . ."

"What happened after you got back to the room—yeah."

My shoulders collapse forward and I drop my head. "I feel terrible about it. I should have handled myself better, I know . . ." I'm channeling the spirit of Scott's words now—about how the impression I give here in this hospital room may be an enduring one. I feel Jill's hand land gently on my back. "But the pacemaker thing is a big deal for me, you know that, and then in the procedure room—Jill, I just . . . It was something out of a horror show and I . . . Well, I shouldn't make excuses."

In the hours since my waking from the procedure—and with the fade-out of lingering sedation—disappointment in myself has become increasingly clear and cutting. I feel suddenly hot—unbearably hot—and sweaty. I push up my sleeves. Wipe my forehead. I exhale, "Shit," leaning forward to pull off my socks.

"Hey, come on now. What's done is done. Let's leave it for now. We've got three days to figure out the handle-yourself-better stuff." She takes the socks from my hands and puts them on the night table.

"Thank you. Yes. Okay, all right . . ." I pull my shoulders back and take a deep breath, trying to reset my composure as quickly as possible. I want to show Jill that she hasn't just walked into three days of taking care of a basket case, but her gaze remains leery. "How you're looking at me right now—it's like you've seen a ghost. It's that bad, huh?"

"Want the truth?"

"I guess so."

"Okay. You're . . . gray."

"My skin, right? I can see it in my toes too—grayish, no oxygen in them . . ." I kick the blanket away from my legs so Jill can see.

"Oh no, no, no . . ." One glance and she's ashen, with her fingertips pressed against her lips. Jill has always been quick to nausea. "Oh, Ames . . . I'm sorry . . . you know how I get . . ." Steadying herself on the armrest of a chair, she flashes a wry smile and jokes, "Who's the patient here, right?" She feigns a lurch toward the nurse call button.

"Code vomit!" I call out.

We break into giggles. I maneuver my legs back into hiding undercover, bringing Jill instant relief.

She straightens up and puts her hands on her hips. "Okay—let's see . . ." Pivoting in a circle, she begins assessing the space around us. I explain that I'd been down the hall in a much smaller room earlier today, but then this L-shaped one opened up near the nurses' station and became mine—"because I'm in for the long haul."

"Uh, yeah . . ." Jill has spotted something that carries her focus and her feet across the floor. "So we're going to have to do something about these . . ." She's over by the window now, gesturing with her hands like the models we watched on The Price Is Right back in junior high. "These cannot stay."

"I'm sure we're not allowed to take down the drapes, Jill."

Her eyebrows wiggle. "You going to need light in here—and a few style touches. I'm going to do a little redecorating. What can I use?" She sets out on a hunt for something to spruce up the bulky curtains. The pall from the long day begins to lift as she sweeps through the room in curious pursuit, searching in the small closet, then heading into the interior bathroom, picking up impractical items for commentary and comic relief as she goes along. "How might we use *this*?" An arm thrusts out of the open bathroom door to show me.

"That's a pee-pee measurer. I have to keep track of my output all day, and then the nurse records it."

"Delightful! And now I think I'll give my hands a good washing, tra-la-la . . . count to fifteen!" I hear a blast of water from the faucet. "Or, better, I'll sing the chorus of a song that fits the occasion—*Ah, ah, ah, ah, stayin' alive, stayin' alive . . . ah, ah, ah, ah . . .*"

She's got me laughing.

"Hey, look! An accessory!" She's found a roll of white medical tape. "Now watch this." Drape by drape—there are four in all—Jill fashions sturdy pull-backs so the heavy curtains at once take on a more tailored look and reveal a much larger expanse of window. "So, tomorrow, there'll be sun."

"*Annie*. Seventh grade musical," I say.

"Remember my red curly wig? *Just thinkin' about. . . to-mor-row . . . clears away the cobwebs and—*"

"Hey, spare me that awful song—I've got a heart condition, ya know!"

"*—the sorrow . . .'til there's none. . .*"

"You're killin' me here . . ." I say, loving the silliness. We're being our goofy selves, and everything about it feels natural—even in this fraught setting. So does the redecorating; Jill has been my design guru for just about every couch, chair, and table in my house, so I welcome her bringing a stylish eye to my hospital home.

"Now, where are we going to put this cot?" Moving on from the curtains, Jill turns her attention to the folded twin-size bed on wheels that's pushed up against the wall. I suggest that she place it parallel to my bed, but she tells me that's all wrong. "The space wants it to be perpendicular," she says, placing her hands on her hips before reaching down for the metal frame. She swings one end of the cot toward my toes and points the other out toward a large window. "I'm going to wish I didn't pull back those curtains when the sun wakes me in the morning."

"The sun won't wake you, don't worry. Dr. Lunchbox will—at around six thirty."

"Doctor *who?*"

I launch into a quick overview of today's doctor encounters while Jill steps back into the bathroom to wash up. It's almost eleven, and we agree it's time for sleep. Soon we're both tucked into our single beds, each in our flannel PJs; it could almost feel like a girls' sleepover, just us two, except for the nurse's aide who comes in to check my pee count and blood pressure.

"Lachalle, this is my friend Jill."

"Hi, Jill! It's so nice of you to stay here with Miss Amy tonight."

"Jill's my oldest friend," I tell her.

"Yeah, I'm eighty-five!"

"You don't look eighty-five to me," Lachalle says, smiling broad and sweet as she secures a blood pressure cuff around my arm. "No talking for a few seconds, please, ladies." The cuff inflates, and I watch the BP numbers on the monitor screen—down, down, down they fall, until the final reading appears: 80/52. "That's pretty low, my dear."

"Can you please take it again?" I say, and then turn to at Jill. "And this time, why don't you tell me that Casey is totally goofing off, not lining up a summer job like I told him . . ."

Lachalle presses the auto-inflate button, and Jill starts in, "What summer job? Casey's gonna just chillax at home—sleep all day, raid your refrigerator, play video games on your living room couch and stain it with orange Cheetos dust . . ."

The blood pressure reading appears for the second time: 90/60.

"See? A few frustrating words about my kid and up it goes!" Lachalle and Jill chuckle just a little, more relieved than amused.

"Lookin' good, so I'll say good night to you ladies." Lachalle turns off the lights on her way out.

Jill opens her iPad. It's time to send an email to the girls; she begins to type while checking content with me. "So you want me to say . . . pacemaker because of slow pulse, and you're staying in the hospital until you get a heart . . . and this is good because you'll move higher on the waiting list, but bad because you don't want to be in the hospital . . ."

"And bad because I don't want a friggin' pacemaker in my heart."

"Yeah, you've always dreaded getting one of those. But can I just ask you—and don't get mad at me, okay—what's so bad about a pacemaker? My impression, and I could be wrong, is that people live just fine with 'em."

"Even if that's true, it doesn't bring me any comfort. I'm afraid of what this thing's going to do to me. My heart is really sick . . . anything could set it off."

"You think they'd put a pacemaker in you if there was going to be a real problem with it?"

"Yes."

"Because why?"

"Because they don't know."

"I have to believe your Cedars doctor knows what he's doing. Isn't he, like, *the* major heart transplant guy?"

"It doesn't matter—these doctors don't have more of a clue than I do when it comes to this stuff. Dr. Kobashigawa is just guessing."

She rolls her eyes. "Ames, come on . . ."

"Come on what? Remember a couple of months ago—Dr. Davis upped one of my heart medicines? It was a tiny little increase because my heartbeat was getting crazier and crazier, remember? And then remember how I wound up in an ambulance that night because my body went rubbery and I felt like I was going to black out—had to slide down the staircase on my butt and lie there on the floor while Scott called 9-1-1?"

She remembers.

"And when I asked Dr. Davis why that happened, he said sorry, must have been too much medicine—you never can tell with a transplanted heart. The same thing happened a few years ago when he tried to put me on a beta-blocker—my heart flipped. We had to call an ambulance again. And he said something like, *Transplanted hearts don't always do so well with beta-blockers.*"

"I see where you're going with this . . ."

"There's just no way for things to go nice and smooth with these wires inside my heart. It's too unpredictable, and I'm frightened of the pacemaker leading to disaster."

Jill goes silent. I shift to the right side of the bed to try to catch her expression, but I can't make it out in the dim iPad glow. She turns to face me straight on and says, "None of us can really know how it is to be you, Ames."

I should have expected it.

This has long been Jill's fallback line; it's her way of bowing out when the commonly held beliefs that healthy people rely on are at odds with my experiences. This line is more useful to both of us here tonight than ever: neither agree nor disagree—take a neutral stance. If the common objective is movement toward a donor heart, then avoidance of confrontation can only help the time pass faster.

"Want to finish this up?" She returns to the email. "Should I just say, *Amy is really upset about having a pacemaker. She's afraid of what it might do to her?*"

"Let's leave that out for now, okay?"

"Okay. I'm just going to add here at the end that the cot's pretty comfortable, but the floor's cold. Lauren's next on the schedule, so I'll tell her to bring slippers. And . . . we're done! Can I send?"

"Sure, thanks."

"Good night, then, Ames."

I turn on my left side and check the monitor before closing my eyes: pulse rate is 113. "Good night."

SOMETHING WAKES ME. It's that ominous heaviness again—like gravity is a deathly pull on my body.

"Jill?"

She's asleep.

"Jill!"

"Wha . . . wha . . . are you okay?" She pops up from her cot.

"I'm sinking . . ."

There's a rustle of sheets and blankets, "What? What do you mean?" She's already up and standing beside my bed.

"There it is, look." I point to the monitor. "The blue number—that's my pulse." *90 . . . 86 . . . 82 . . . 79 . . . 76 . . .*

Jill's contact lenses are out; she's rifling around for her glasses when, all of a sudden, pain blazes through my arms and up toward my neck.

"*Ow, ow, ow, ow!*" I cry out, gasping.

"What is it! What's happening!"

"There's burning! Down my arms, through my back."

"What should I do?" She is standing over me now, blinking rapidly.

"I don't know!" What I'm feeling is nothing like a muscle ache or even a spasm; it's more a deep scorching of my insides, as if my blood were aflame and singeing my veins from the inside out. I'm desperate to be distracted from it, immediately in need of sensation that might counter the agony.

I writhe, collapsing forward. The pain has taken over my chest now. "Will you rub my shoulders?" I plead. I don't really expect that this or any sort of touch will have the power to halt whatever is happening physiologically, but I need something soothing to focus on. Jill presses her fingertips into my back, but it's too much. "No, no, not good. That's worse. Uh, just . . . maybe just scratch—gently, gently. Ah, it's too painful."

She switches at once to a feathery sweep across my back.

I glance up at the monitor and exhale a whispery "Oh no": My heart rate seems to be stuck at 76. "Something's really wrong here. If my pulse drops below eighty, the pacemaker's supposed to kick in—that's what the doctor told me."

"Maybe . . . uh . . . *that's* what you're feeling?" She turns her head again and again toward the monitor.

"It's not . . . *ow* . . . supposed to be . . . *ow, ow* . . . painful, I don't think. And why isn't the damn thing working? It should surge my heartbeat right up . . ."

"You want me to get the nurse? Or . . . or . . . do you want me to stay? Tell me what . . . what . . . to do . . ." Jill's lips are trembling now.

I grab her wrist. "The nurse, yeah, go get the nurse. Or the resident, if you see him. Young guy. Black hair. Baird or something . . ."

"Okay, just hold on, hold on . . . I'll be back in two seconds." Jill dashes into the hallway in her flannels. I pull my knees up to my chest and wrap my arms around them, rocking back and forth, whispering, "You're okay, you're okay . . ."

The lights come on. Dr. Lunchbox hurries in, saying, "I hear you're having pain."

"Yes. Started when my pulse dropped. Crazy burning. Unbearable."

"Pains that bad, huh? Well, the telemetry would have alerted me if you were having a heart attack." Jill's hands fly to her cheeks. She clears her throat to catch my attention and asks me silently—*Call Scotty?* I shake my head—*No.* The doctor continues, "Your pacemaker shouldn't let your pulse get below eighty." He gazes at the monitor for a few long seconds.

"It's not doing its thing . . ." I say.

"Actually, it is. I can see it pacing on the EKG up there. You heart's just not responding."

"Why?"

"I don't know. Maybe Dr. Kobashigawa can . . . oop! There she goes now." *80 . . . 83 . . . 87 . . .* "Any better?"

The pain subsides instantly. "Yeah . . . look at that . . . yeah."

Jill begins to pace the floor, shaking tension from her arms and hands. "Phew, phew . . ."

"Is this thing supposed to kill like all hell every time it fires, Dr. Baird?" I ask.

"No. I'll put in a request for the pacemaker team to stop by in the morning. Maybe they can readjust your voltage."

My voltage? Yuck . . .

"I'm here all night if you need anything. Should I turn off the lights on my way out?"

"Thanks, Doctor, yes."

Jill moves shakily to her cot and slips under the blanket.

"Well, that sucked," I say.

"Sure scared *me.*"

"I guess we should try to get some sleep."

Jill's voice goes high-pitched. "Oh, sure. That'll be a b-breeze. I couldn't f-feel more relaxed right n-now!" Her lips are trembling, still.

"Good times . . . good times . . ." I kid.

"Oh, yeah . . ."

Sarcastic banter brings no comfort this time. Fear is ours to share now, no longer mine alone to feel its toss and turn through the night. My trauma is not merely witnessed in this room. A friend's presence bears its haunting along with me.

I close my eyes and settle into sleep with one thought: *Jill's here, Jill's here, Jill's here . . .*

From: Jill Dawson
Subject: Amy
Date: April 2, 2014 at 6:52 PM
To: Ann Burrell, Lauren Steale, Jane Keller, Leja Babic, Valerie Yablon, Jody Solomon, Robin Adelson, Joy Ceterra

Hi Everyone,

As Jody wrote to all of you last night, the procedure to insert the pacemaker was more complicated than expected. Here's a bit more about what happened—Amy told me that the doctor was very rough with her, the nurses did nothing to comfort or talk to her—and, ultimately, the doctor required that Amy be sedated in order to finish the procedure. She is really upset about how rough the doctor was with her physically, angry at the nurses for not once taking her hand or asking how she was doing, and mad at herself for "letting" the doctor put her under—she imagines that countless errors were made while she was under and that, although she may not remember what happened, her body will never forget the "trauma" of the doctor's "brutality" (her words).

I tell you this because Amy is extremely upset and her anger will be peppered into any communication with her. She is understandably exhausted, physically and emotionally, and seems to have exceeded her capacity to deal with all of this.

It's a tough situation all around. If you want to reach out to Amy, best just to keep it short, via email or text, tell her you love her and are thinking about her. I don't know how much energy she has to respond—so don't be surprised if you don't get a response. I'm going to try to get some sleep now . . . xo

At the sun's first light, Lachalle rolls a stand-up scale into my room and parks it beside my bed. She sees that I'm already up. "Good morning, Amy. I need to get your weight."

"Can I skip it?" I whisper, hoping not to wake Jill.

"I have to write it over there on the wall so the doctors can see." She points to a dry-erase board in my direct line of vision: *My weight today is____.*

"You're not serious . . ."

She nods. "Every morning."

"Oh, come on—no . . . *no* . . ." My eyes dart from the scale to the door and back again.

The idea of looking at my weight all day sets me on a panicky edge. Before arriving at Cedars, I hadn't gotten on a scale in years. Fitting into the same pair of jeans had always been a sufficient indicator of whether my weight has remained within a general range. But when I got to the ER, I was already eight pounds heavier than I had been a few days prior, as my heart is no longer strong enough to pump excess fluid from my body. To me, weight gain signifies an alarming medical condition. And a dry-erase marker number on my wall would serve as yet another visceral, daily reminder of my powerlessness against heart failure.

I tell Lachalle that my weight scares the hell out of me, that's all.

Jill speaks up: "I think I might have an idea." She's awake but groggy, still on her back and under the sheet and blanket. She flips to her belly and thinks for a few seconds. "How about if you get on the scale and face *away* from the number?"

"I guess I can do that. And I don't want to cause you any trouble, Lachalle. You're so nice to put up with my nuttiness . . . I know you have to roll on to the next room . . . but take a look, get a load of these puffball feet!" I pull my legs from under the blanket and hang them off the side of the bed. "I have Fred Flintstone ankles too, *yabba dabba doo.*" I step onto the scale.

Lachalle tells me I'm a funny one and records the number on a notepad. "You ladies can go back to sleep now. See you tonight."

Jill's already drifting off. I reach back to fluff the two pillows behind me, hoping to join her for another hour of sleep before a doctor comes in, but something catches my eye. I groan to myself, "Oh, well, that's just great!"

I don't even realize I've spoken aloud until Jill replies, "What's that?"

"Lachalle wrote my weight on the wall. What's the point of turning away from the scale if she's going to post it right in front of me?"

Jill sits up and rubs her eyes.

"I'm one twenty-three! I was one twenty yesterday. One thirteen a week ago."

"You said it yourself, it's the fluid. Your heart can't pump it out of—"

"It's just hard to look a ten-pound weight gain in the face, knowing what it means."

"Okay, all right . . ." She gets up from her cot and plods into the bathroom—"Let's try something"—then emerges a minute later, smiling, with a sheet of paper towel folded into a perfect square. "How about this?" Using the roll of medical tape from last night, she creates a flap to cover the number on the dry-erase board. "Pen?" she asks, and I pass her one from my night table: *See weight here*, she writes on the paper square. "The doctor can just lift it up."

"It's perfect, but—"

"You want me to put a small piece of tape at the bottom too."

"No, you've done enough already. Gosh, Jill . . ."

I'm thankful for her swift solution. I'm not a child, and yet what Jill has just done to soothe my angst is the same sort of loving magic we both performed many times as mothers when our kids were young: we found ways to address their concerns, no matter how irrational. Sometimes a small light that threw a night sky on the wall through moon and star cutouts was enough to calm them. Other times, it took a line of Matchbox cars across the bottom of a closet door to keep the boogeyman at bay. We had to be patient, creative, and quick on our feet to quiet the fears we couldn't quite explain away to our little ones. There would come a time, though, when the piles of stuffed animals on the bed no longer allowed sufficient space to fit the much bigger body sleeping among them. There would come a time for a reality prompt while tucking in a twelve-year-old among the teddies, a nudge to let go of childish anxieties: "Something's got to change here, don't you think?" we'd say, trusting that he'd figure it out.

And now here's Jill, prodding me to find a more appropriate approach to my current environment. "I have to say this," she begins. "I think you'd want me to point it out." She's not sliding back into bed this time, but rather launching into the motions of morning, pulling a toothbrush out of her toiletry bag. She sits beside me and continues, "This weight thing. The giant-ankles thing. You've got to find a better way to, uh, express yourself, let's put it that way. One twenty-three— it's just *not* a lot of weight, I'm sorry. I bet Lachalle wishes she was one twenty-three. Hey, I wouldn't mind weighing that myself."

I shift my eyes away—embarrassed.

"And your ankles. Take a look at mine . . ." She throws her leg up on the bed and lifts her pajama bottom. "This is without any heart failure fluid going on!"

Her ankle is pretty darn slender, but I still get the point.

"I'm not saying I wouldn't get hung up on gaining ten pounds in a week," she adds. "I'm just saying that you don't want to sound like a kook." Her eyebrows arch sharp with expectation.

My conscience twists; I look down at my nails. I don't know what to say. Direct, uninvited criticism is something Jill and I have doled out fairly regularly as mothers of teenagers—but not as friends. If we've learned lessons from each other in the past, the mechanism has been subtler. But here in my hospital room, there's an urgency to it. I need to reflect on my behavior *now*—and change it. Jill means to help me . . .

"Morning, morning!" Dr. Kobashigawa interrupts my contemplation, striding into the room. He's fresh and energetic in a starched white coat and daisy-dot tie. Jill shoots me a look—*Should I go?*

I pop my eyes—*Stay.*

He shakes my hand, pulls up a chair, and sits down. "All right, all right. Well, Dr. Baird told me a bit about what happened last night."

"Yeah, this pacemaker—wow. It was rough."

"Yes. Well, let me share with you why it is so important that you have one in place right now . . ." My heart is so sick and weak, he explains, that it wants to stop beating; this is the reason for my dropping pulse. And when my heartbeat spirals down this way, the doctor warns, all my organs—kidneys, liver, lungs, brain—are deprived of the fuel they need to perform their functions. Jill is taking notes.

"That's why you've got so much fluid on board. Your kidneys can't do their work without a good supply of oxygen." He looks at me directly with dark, earnest eyes, and pulls the left side of his white coat over the right, leaning forward into an ever so slight bow. He does this again. And once more, still. There's serenity in his movements, a sense of ritual that calms me. I feel myself staring at a pin on his coat.

"You like my pin, I see . . . It represents the number of heart transplants we did last year—one hundred nineteen."

I snap back from my admiring stupor. "Columbia did only sixty-three when I had mine in back in the eighties."

"The old days, ah, yes. You're a trailblazer, Amy. You should feel very proud of how well you've done. It's inspiring." He pauses and becomes very still, making sure I absorb the compliment. It feels to me like Dr. K is aware that any pride I might have felt in achieving long-term survival has now been eclipsed by the utter failure of my heart. "That's right, yes . . ." he confirms, meeting my eyes.

I feel my cheeks flush—I like this guy.

I like the way he shook my hand.

I like the soft rasp in his voice, the daisy tie, the way he holds his arms across his middle after finishing a series of coat pulls.

"So, we've set your pacemaker at eighty to make reasonably sure your heart is fueling your organs."

"But it wasn't working last night."

He chuckles. "It was working fine, actually . . ." The problem, he says, is that my heart is having trouble responding because the pacemaker isn't positioned ideally. It seems Dr. Wayne had a devil of a time during the implantation; he couldn't find a workable spot to anchor the pacemaker. "Your atrium is so riddled with disease, the wires wouldn't hold. Dr. Wayne could only attach it to your ventricle . . . and even this didn't give him many options for placement. Your vasculopathy is quite extensive." He pauses, stroking his chin. "Quite."

And this, he goes on to explain, is the reason for the terrible pain when my pulse plunged last night. The pacemaker was firing—or, as the doctor put it, *pacing*—but its mechanism could only activate the ventricle, not the atrium. The result was that some of my heart valves failed to open for the sudden blood flow propelled by the pacemaker's activation. When blood is forced through tight spaces (like what happens in people with severely blocked arteries), it causes what is commonly thought of as a heart attack symptom: excruciating, stabbing, fiery pain. Closed valves during pacing will trigger this kind of pain every time my pacemaker fires.

"This is why we need to get you a heart as soon as possible," Dr. Kobashigawa says. "We're working on moving you to a 1A designation on the waiting list."

Jill sighs with relief.

"1A means a life expectancy of about two weeks," I tell her.

"She's a smart one, she is!" he chirps, but turns immediately serious. "Yes, that's true of 1A. The pacemaker is intended to prevent that outcome. But if your heart failure continues to worsen exponentially as it has over the last couple of weeks, I worry that the pacemaker won't help." Dread clutches my stomach—it's not good when a doctor says, *I worry.* Jill puts her pen down.

"This is why we're filing papers with UNOS to make you 1A as soon as possible," Dr. Kobashigawa concludes, rising from his chair. "Mind if I examine you for a minute?"

"All right."

He begins by assessing the prominent, purplish vein on the right side of my neck. It's called the jugular, and the higher its protrusion stretches toward my ear, the more dangerous the underlying heart failure. "Impressive," he says aloud. "I'd like to show young Dr. Baird— you're a great teaching tool."

Next, it's the stethoscope; Dr. K presses the chest piece alongside my sternum and places his other hand on my left shoulder simultaneously —a two-handed maneuver that comforts me with its tenderness; my New York transplant doctor's technique has always been one-handed, as if pushing me and my dreadful heart away. "Ah, it's so easy to hear your gallop. Remarkable."

This is terrible praise, of course. Neck veins aren't supposed to bulge blue and straight up to the earlobe. And a healthy heartbeat shouldn't gallop.

Impressive. Remarkable. Jill may find hope in these words or hear them as accolades at first blush, but they turn my skin clammy with anxiety—because I know their dark significance instantly. When a doctor listens to your heart, what you want is a quick recitation of adjectives like *normal* or *unremarkable*. I shoot Jill a side-glance and notice that her demeanor is more relaxed now. She's understandably swayed by the casual timbre of Dr. K's voice and the false positives of his language. As Jill sees it, we're just having a frank but very calm and oddly pleasant little chat here, the three of us.

I realize I've forgotten to introduce her by name. "This is my friend Jill, by the way."

"Excuse my pajamas," she says.

"Nah, it's all good, it's all good. Very nice to meet you. You're a wonderful friend to be here for Amy." He extends his hand to her, and then to me, for a parting shake. "Tomorrow, then."

We watch him turn to leave, our eyes glued to the back of his white coat as it glides away from us. He opens the door with one hand while pressing the wall-mounted hand sanitizer with the other, exiting in a swift, seamless motion that delivers him into the hallway without a post-Purell touch of the door handle—and he's gone.

Jill fans herself with her hand. "Wow."

SIX SOUTH IS a sprawling rectangle—a wide, immaculate expanse of bright tiled straightaways lined with patients' rooms and leading to corners where folded cots for guests stand at the ready. There's art, some of it original and signed, including a few numbered prints by Lichtenstein. Oxygen tanks, tall and forest green, pop up at intervals, some of them on wheeled bases alongside defibrillator carts covered loosely with clear plastic tarps. The occasional doctor stands at a hallway computer station. Nurses traverse noiselessly, as if on tiptoe, their pathways set by purpose, some of them talking to themselves while they count a fistful of tubes or multiple IV fluid bags in different sizes. Their patients have failing hearts, and most—as Jill and I can see through the open doors as we walk the hall now—are gray and hollowed out, tongues hanging from their mouths, which prompts Jill to designate them O's or Q's (nomenclature she learned from her father, a now re-tired physician). "O's show no tongue and Q's have it out to the side, like this." She shows me and I smile, not because I find it amusing, but because I'm thankful that Jill is still able to see me as separate from my floor mates here at Cedars. And maybe she's got a point: it's ten a.m., prime stroll time for patients, and I'm the only one taking on the large square hallway this morning.

"Good for you, up and walking!" a nurse calls out as she passes, lift-ing her fist toward the ceiling to cheer me on. I smile and wave.

"*Look at us, we're walking . . .*" Jill sings out of the side of her mouth. It's Jerry Lewis's theme song for that muscular dystrophy telethon we grew up watching year after year. Here in the hospital hallway, it strikes me as a little sad at first: my walking pace today is disabled in its own right. But the way Jill stretches her lips from end to end, crooning like a Jerry Lewis ventriloquist, well—I'm going to giggle, even if it steals my breath.

"I need to stop a second, whoa." I can't laugh and walk at the same time. We turn the corner and I reach for the handrail on the wall. "Dis-tract me," I urge—*inhale, exhale, inhale, exhale . . .*

She dives into chatter about her son. "I thought you'd never ask. Let's talk about Griffen and . . . *college*! We're coming up with some possible schools, planning some visits. I've got the list—a whole folder, actually—back in the room. I am going to need a lot of help from you when application time comes, so you gotta stick around, if you know what I mean. That sounds selfish . . ." She pauses, adding sarcasm, "*Is that selfish of me?*" Jill is up in her soprano range now, hitting that high C like she did when she chirped *college* a few seconds ago. But I know her asking is partly serious.

We start walking again and come upon an elderly patient holding tight to a nurse. The back of his hospital gown shifts and parts as he steps forward, revealing the backs of two deconditioned thighs and a slice of naked, sagging buttocks—right cheek, left cheek, right cheek, left. We catch up quickly and pass him by.

"You're still beatin' the ninety-year-olds," Jill says.

"Yeah, but he's wearing fall-risk socks. It's not a fair competition." I've refused the fluorescent-yellow ankle socks that were on my bed along with a Cedars toiletry kit when I was admitted two nights ago. They have a sticky underside designed for patients who are unstable and at risk for falling. When the nurse asked me if my fall-risk socks were the right size, I knew I'd never wear them. I relay this now to Jill, telling her that I'll always put on sneakers before stepping into the hall, even if I have to stop and catch my breath after reaching down to tie them.

She turns around to get another look at the yellow-footed man and shrugs. "They're pretty cool socks, actually."

"Put those on and it's the walk of shame—or doom," I say. "Why don't they call them 'comfy treads'—something without a suggestion of landing on your ass, maybe? I don't get it. And even this over here," I say, pointing to a sign affixed to the wall where, again, I've had to stop to relieve the gasping. "As if this doesn't make patients feel like shit . . ."

Just then, Jody emerges from the elevator vestibule a few feet ahead. "Ames! Jill!" She's full of pep—probably went to a spin class at six a.m., showered, dressed, and now she's out and about in casual Jody attire of jeans, sandals, and a flattering tunic-style blouse. "So good to see you, Jill, it's been a long time. You look great!"

"You too! How are the girls?"

"Rachel just got a great internship, and Emily's at . . ."

They chat. I breathe.

Jody's holding a cup of coffee, buzzing with delight over having two New York friends in her neighborhood at once. "I thought I'd visit for a few hours this morning," she tells me. I didn't expect Jody to show up this soon, if at all, given the way I acted in front of her after the pacemaker implantation yesterday. "And I'd love to come tomorrow too, but I already know I've got a case. I can be here Thursday and Friday and Saturday morning, though, with Jack . . ."

"What's the case?" Jill asks. "I didn't know you were working these days."

"Part-time. Doing some nonprofit legal stuff. I advocate in the schools for kids with disabilities and make sure they get all the services they're entitled to. Shall we walk?" We start again slowly, three of us in a row, taking up a good portion of the hallway.

"I was just pointing this out to Jill," I say, stepping away from the wall so Jody can see the shiny white sign mounted on a five-foot horizontal stretch of black background: *We have a passion for Heart Failure!*

Jody opens her mouth and stares in wide-eyed silence for a few seconds as her geniality clashes with the dissonant strike of the words in front of us. But within seconds, she lets loose: "Can you believe this? A *passion?* For *heart failure?* I mean, I'm all for loving your work, but there are other ways to say it, like maybe, *We're passionate about caring for our patients.*"

"Even the words *heart failure,*" I add, "it's a medical term, I get that. But when it describes a hospital area, like, with a big sign, it can make patients feel bad when they go there."

Jody tilts her head. "How's that, Ames?"

"What I mean is, if there's a place where heart patients go for care and it's called, say, a *heart failure clinic,* it makes everyone in there a failure by definition. I know, not literally, but, hey, would you like the word *failure* assigned to you? Oh, but no offense intended, it's only your freakin' *heart* that's a failure . . ."

Jill and Jody laugh in agreement, but I can feel myself getting heated. To them it's only semantics, but it bothers me deeply, just like the idea of the fall-risk socks. Because when you take on the names, places, and even devices assigned to your illness, you start to believe in them and, eventually, become them. These things I say and do that make my friends laugh nervously or lift their eyebrows in awkward discontent—they're spitfire signs of my refusal to be swallowed up by the failure that pumps deep within my chest. And as I see it, they've been central to my longevity against heart transplant odds.

But tenacity isn't pretty—not the way I do it, anyway. Holding tight to life means correcting misconceptions that would weaken me, even if this means confronting doctors head-on with choice words. In this way, I laced into the cardiologist who first pronounced me a *sick girl* when I was twenty-four and didn't yet understand that my heart problem was serious (I pronounced him an idiot and vowed never to refer to myself as he did). This same gritty insistence on survival and strength has also incited me to snap at friends when they suggest that I ask Scott to drag the two large garbage pails up from the bottom of our driveway on collection day instead of struggling up the hill with them myself. My response is so quick to outrage that you'd think they had urged me to give up my car key for lack of mental competence.

It is instances like these, I know, that Scott had in mind as reference points when encouraging me always to be carefully conscious of the tone and content of my words while in California.

Clearly, the fervor with which I brandish the last bits of my well self is not a display everyone is going to applaud. And yet, after decades of fight against cardiac death, I have learned to curse with all my might what I dare not become in body, mind, and spirit: weak, sick, and, worst of all, failed. Ferocity and saltiness have been vital components of my body armor and longevity. One soft step and I'm as *passionate about heart failure* as that sign on the wall.

Never, I tell myself. I'll fight to be passionate about the parts that *aren't* failing me, thanks.

"Tell me, girls, what do you see when you look at this image?" I say, changing tack. We've come upon a framed color print just before making the final turn toward my room. At first glance, the image appears to be a scissor positioned vertically, its rounded handles at the bottom and shears pointing up. We move closer and stand shoulder to shoulder, the three of us, directly in front of it.

"Here's a hint—it's not just a scissor . . ." I'd already figured it out a few days earlier when taking a walk with Jack, although I didn't share my interpretation with him at the time. ". . . It's a penis, right?"

"Yes, I am agree with you!" Leja has come up suddenly from behind. She hands me hot chocolate in a Starbucks cup, pivots to the right, and continues straight on to my hospital room, calling out over her shoulder, "I've got for you clean underwear!"

Jody is bewildered, but not Jill; she's known Leja as long as I have and was my Ikea shopping partner when I was setting up the furnished apartment for her years ago. When we arrive back at the room a minute later, we find Leja wrestling Jill's open cot into a folded, upright position. "We need bigger space. And another chair. See?"

We're standing in the doorway, steering clear of Leja as she heave-hos at whirlwind speed. We can't see the whole of the L-shaped room from where we're standing. A voice calls out to us from within: "I'm here! It's Sidra! The nurse said you were walking. I thought I'd wait."

"Hi, Sidra!" I call back to the guest I cannot see.

Screech, snap! The cot finally submits, and Leja secures the fold with a metal latch. "Now I get chair," she says, charging by us and into the hallway. We enter the room and find a blond woman in a sea-foam green blazer and white pants. She's got a wiry Chihuahua on her lap.

"This is Taj—*say hi, Taj!*—I'm a dog visit volunteer too." She points to the Cedars-Sinai patch on her blazer. "Recognize the uniform?"

She'd been wearing it in the ER when Leja and I arrived there a few nights ago. It was near midnight, and her volunteer shift as patient facilitator was about to end when she decided to reach for one more file. That's when fate, as Sidra called it, kicked in. "I saw your name on the intake form, and the hairs stood up on my arm," she told Leja and me after escorting us to a curtained cubicle deep within the ER.

Indeed, there was eerie coincidence in her happening to be there when I arrived. I'd gotten Sidra's number from a childhood friend I'd spoken to briefly before leaving for LA; she said she knew a volunteer in the ER at Cedars and urged me to give her a call. I planned to do so once things settled down, but emergency beat me to it.

Sidra tells Jill the tale from the night we met, full of excitement. "And then *Jody* walks into the ER to see Amy. What are the odds?" This was the second coincidence: Sidra's husband had worked side by side with Jack early in their careers. "It's spooky, I tell you."

Leja agrees heartily, jumping in with tea-leaf contemplations: "This tells to us something . . ."

My focus drifts as I stroke the bony head of Taj, the far too docile Chihuahua sitting indifferently on my lap. *This dog is no fun at all.*

Jody and Jill start talking among themselves. Jill reaches into her bag and pulls out a folder. "He wants to go to Vanderbilt," she says, "but I'm not sure it's the right place for him . . ."

Taj, you don't care that I'm petting your skinny little back, do you?

"There is reason that you meet Amy, but what it is?" Leja keeps on.

"And I had just spoken to Joni earlier that night!" Sidra howls. "She called to ask if I'd heard from Amy yet! Can you imagine?"

"So I've got Vanderbilt, Michigan, Tufts, Wake Forest, Tulane . . ." Jill tells Jody.

"Yay, Tulane! Rachel and Emily couldn't be happier there . . ."

You're probably loaded with germs, Taj—sick patients putting their hands on you all day. I've got to wash really well after you're off my lap.

LEJA: Is interesting to me what you say, Sidra . . .

SIDRA: I have to just tell you, things like this happen to me all the time. I'm just that kind of person. I've got an energy . . .

JILL: And there's University of Richmond, Boston College, maybe Elon . . .

JODY: You think Griffen will apply early decision, or will he . . .

Chatter. Chatter. Chatter.

I'm surrounded.

Two women on my left.

Two on my right.

And I'm in the middle, on a hospital bed.

Is this how the days will go? Like a coffee klatch after yoga class?

I suppose so.

We can't talk about illness and death all day, can we? I wouldn't want that all day, every day—and my friends couldn't sustain it. But as entrenched as I am in my heart's failing state, everyone who sits by my side here will be rooted in life, life, life—the frivolities and the serious matters, the here and now and the six months from now. *I'm* the odd-ball here. *I'm* the one who's tuned in more to the blue number on the monitor screen than to the surrounding chitchat that's meant to pass my time. How, then, to be good company and a grateful friend to each of these women who come to sit beside me for these difficult hours? And how to help them be the same for me?

I'm not sure yet. I haven't done this before. With my first transplant, only a few friends came to my hospital room during my two-month wait for a donor heart at Columbia. While we supported each other pretty well through boyfriend-breakup tears—armed with tissues and willing to devote a few Sunday morning hours for a Bloody Mary brunch of listening and cajoling—we held only loosely to our friends' grander troubles, taking them on even as we let them slide, sympathizing swiftly but falling short of real empathy. We weren't steadfast. We were girls.

I was as slippery a friend as any at twenty-five. Looking back, I can hardly believe the light touch I gave to what I now see as profound, sad, and even hellish happenings that befell some of my girlfriends in their early twenties. How was it, then, that when a close friend had an abortion at a clinic one morning, I merely showed up casually at her apartment that afternoon? When I rang the bell, another friend answered (she was on her way out), making me think maybe I needn't have come; I was but one in a rotation of many. My friend lay on her bed surrounded by fluffy stuffed animals with tags still attached, boxes of chocolates, and bright helium balloons grazing the ceiling—evidence of gift-bearing visitors come and gone.

I, however, arrived empty-handed—a gaffe that my friend's look of disappointment made clear to me. And I felt bad.

Not that abortions are times for balloons and candy. But what made me question myself—back then and even now—was what I failed to bring into that room in the way of thoughtful presence and intention, or even in the way of gifts that would have been more useful company than the plush polar bear or giant froggy perched on the bed. I walked into that room without anything to give of myself, I realized within seconds, and it grew me up some—right then and there.

Even so, none of us had grown up enough to know how to bring our friendship to bear on my transplant waiting list stay at Columbia just a few years later. Jill trudged up to the northern tip of Manhattan to visit me twice in eight weeks, which was more than any other friend. One time, she arrived all a-sparkle in a blue polka-dot dress, arm in arm with a great-looking boyfriend; they posed like a wedding cake topper at the foot of my bed, smiled through a few sentences, and headed out to a party. For her second visit, she came alone and told me she could stay for a whole hour, so I asked if she'd help me wash my hair; it had been over a month since I stood in a shower. And so began the great chore of holding my head over the sink to wet down, soap up, rinse, and condition my thick, chaotic mess of curly hair—the volume and consistency of which Jill, a silky-straight-tresses gal, had never held in hand, let alone combed through. She struggled, grunted, exhaled in huffs until, finally, she finished and I was back in bed with a towel turban snuggly in place. Jill fell into a chair beside me and said, "That's exhausting! It's like a major arm workout! I never knew you had hair like that . . ."

None of us can really know how it is to be you, Ames . . .

Twenty-five years ago, Jill had no idea how thick and difficult my hair was—until she got really, really close and held its wet weight in her hands. Then she knew; then she really knew.

Maybe this time around, my transplant will move us beyond appearances and into the true tangled mess of it all. The push-pull of life on one side and death on the other might be better conveyed and understood experientially; words are merely heard, but happenings engage all the senses, right? Whatever takes place here in this hospital room, then, may illuminate our disparate stances and beliefs better than my friends or I ever could through years of discussion. Perhaps here and now, all of us will come to appreciate one another's viewpoints in the clearest, brightest light yet. This is my hope. And it is the happiest ending I can think of right now.

SCOTT WAS RIGHT about the importance of taking other people's feelings into account. I know this because I find myself looking now at the back of Jill's head. She's turned away from me, and I don't expect a change of position anytime soon. It was only two hours ago that all seemed fine. Then, something shifted in me: Jill was typing tonight's email report on her iPad, and I left her to it—or, rather, got upset suddenly and told her, "Just write it yourself, I don't care," before stomping out of the room and into the hallway, where I hid (yes, *hid*) in a remote waiting room. The lights had been turned off hours ago, but a small TV remained on, mounted high in the corner, so I sat in front of it and looked up at Lakers and Clippers darting across the screen.

It was the sunset that did it. It cut through the pleasant distractions of the day and confronted me with the night to come. I know my pulse will inevitably slow at night and cause the pacemaker to fire . . . I know the pain is inevitable . . . and I feel trapped.

We had decided to put on mud masks, Jill and I, about twenty minutes before I ran out on her. When our faces were fully covered, Lachalle came in for a blood pressure check and declared the scene "spa night," telling us we're plenty pretty enough already and that she hopes her skin looks as good as ours when she's fifty. We took selfies, and I sent one to Dr. Davis back in New York, a goof that Jill encouraged: *Look what happens when you get a pacemaker*, I wrote just below my muddy green face. *What do you mean?* he wrote back a few minutes later, sending Jill and me into guffaws. "He can't be serious!" she said. "With his fancy socks and that earring hole—who *is* this guy!" She'd come with me to an appointment with Dr. Davis just before I left for LA and, in typical Jill fashion, emerged with observations I hadn't noticed in twenty-five years of encountering this man. "You saw his socks, right?" she said. "Striped like the Wicked Witch of the West. The guy's going for a bit of style, I'll give him that. And did you notice the earring hole on his left side? He's got a past! Dr. Davis—cool guy, or nerd with high aspirations?"

We concluded here tonight that he's just plain inscrutable, but not before we had a few more laughs—imitating his toneless, dry delivery of medical conclusion: "Your. Heart. Is. Uh. Failing." It sounded funny to us now, *ha-ha-ha* . . .

We washed off the masks and got into our beds—Jill with her iPad and me with my sick heart. And that's when I felt like I had to get the hell out of there.

It wasn't Jill's fault. She hadn't left my room all day for more than a few bathroom breaks, not even taking time to step out and get herself some fresh air when Scott came or when Jack showed up with a big cup of Carvel after dinner. She was kind and watchful and loving. We'd figured out how to get through a whole day and night together in one room, with pee-pee measuring and dog visits, pulse drops and back rubs, slow hallway walks and college-list brainstorming. We were spreadsheet pioneers, staking out the route for those to follow, even with the undercurrent of rattling realities like cardiogenic shock. We managed to establish a comfortable groove of sorts.

And yet, I ran.

Or, really, I marched with intensity—out of my room, without warning, without apology. What she didn't know was that my mind had started whirling when the sky turned dusky pink, and that by the time we turned out the lights a few hours later, my thoughts were near explosion. And then they blew.

Here comes the agony . . . I can't stop it . . .

I sat in the dim, deserted waiting room, vowing to keep my pajama-clad butt there for two hours, damn it, even though the chair was uncomfortable and the glow from the TV threw an eerie shadow across the unmanned reception desk. It meant something to me to still have the decision to walk out of my hospital room within my full control, one action of body and mind that I could carry out without anyone's help or permission, one choice that was not made for me a priori just because the alternative was death. With this self-imposed sit-in, I wrangled free will for a couple of hours. But, at the same time, I felt regret bubbling up inside me for not simply saying to Jill, *I can't focus on the email right now. I'm having a hard time getting into bed because I know the pain is coming. I need to be alone for a little while and shore myself up for it.* I knew that communicating more openly could have landed me in this same chair, but without spewing hurt. Why then—*really*—did I choose to do otherwise?

As I sat there ruminating, the frustrated angst that had seized me in my hospital room took a sharp turn inward. I imagined Jill sitting on her cot, bewildered and hurt. Digging uncomfortably deep into my motives, I asked myself whether part of my aim in fleeing Jill was to make her feel bad.

Was it? I demanded an answer then and there. *Did the atmosphere of the evening become unbearably upbeat, with mud masks and selfies too soon after the cath lab ordeal?*

No, that wasn't it . . . it was more, um . . . uh . . .

Yes. That *was* it.

Remorse led to tears, and then to full-on weeping. *I'm so sorry, I lost myself, I have to be stronger, kinder. I've got to find a better way to express my emotions, just like Scott said . . .*

And then Lachalle found me.

She put her hand on my shoulder. "What're you doin' there? You're feeling kinda sad, aren't ya. Your friend's worried about you." It had been over an hour since I'd left the room.

"I'm watching the Clippers-Lakers game," I lied. "And yeah, I'm really sad. My doctor gave me some bad news this morning."

"Hard to wait for a heart, it sure is. How 'bout coming on back to your room? I know you want to be nice to your nice friend . . ."

Be nice to my friend.

I'm not being nice to my friend.

My best friend.

Who rushed out of work and flew across the country to see me.

My friend who laid hands on my back last night, soothing me through the pain—so completely present, so vigilant, making sure that I did not for one minute feel alone.

"You're lucky to have a friend like that here with you. So many patients on this floor, they don't have people."

I'd noticed this while walking this morning with Jill; peeking through open doors at the O's and Q's, we saw there were no visitors inside any of these rooms, no flowers, no photos taped to the wall or cheerful cards on the night table. "So sad," we said to each other, putting an end to the O/Q game. But something struck our sympathies even deeper when we turned the second corner: a hunched, wrinkled woman slumped in a chair just outside the entrance to her room, looking around hopefully as if in a porch rocker on Main Street where she might get the chance to chat up a neighbor passing by. Yet she took no interest in our *hello* and *good morning*. Maybe she was waiting for the frail old man in the yellow fall socks? Wouldn't it be great if they found each other?

I stood up and Lachalle slipped her arm through mine, buddy-style. "Good choice. You make me glad," she said, and we strolled together through the late-night hallways of Six South.

Back in the room now, Jill is already in her cot and facing the wall. The iPad is turned off. I suppose the email has been sent; I gave her my okay, after all.

"Jill?"

She doesn't budge.

Oh no . . .

Scott's advice was crucial. It all comes down to how I want to live these days: I can try to force a deeper, more painful understanding of the situation on everyone around me (generating more alienation than empathy, it seems). Or I can find a way to love and be loved here in this hospital room. The time is not for forcing upon every friend who sits beside me the truth of what she could never quite understand before. My mistakes with first Jody and now Jill tell me this loud and clear. The time, as it turns out, is for good-byes.

Cardiogenic shock . . . galloping disease progression . . . neck vein worthy of a medical tutorial . . .

I look up at the blue number on the monitor—112. Then I close my eyes and speak to the turned back I can't bear to see. "You're the best friend any girl could hope for."

No answer.

I slide under the covers and bring them all the way up to my chin, but there's no hiding from the lesson of this night.

Friends—even best ones—have limits.

I must do better.

From: Jill Dawson
Subject: Amy
Date: April 3, 2014 at 3:56 PM
To: Ann Burrell, Lauren Steale, Jane Keller, Valerie Yablon, Jody Solomon, Robin Adelson, Joy Ceterra, Leja Babic

When I left LA early this morning, Amy was sleeping soundly. She had an ok night, up many times with chest/arm pain when the pacemaker had to kick in to keep her heart rate up. Her spirits were pretty good throughout the night—and, with all of you amazing visitors lined up for the coming weeks, and the uplifting presence of the West Coast steadies (Jody and Leja), here's to hoping they will stay that way.

My time with Amy and Scotty was precious—we had some great laughs, and tears, some very honest talks and many long spaces of quiet. Just praying that a heart is coming soon. It's an exhausting wait.

Some advice re. sleeping at the hospital: Amy usually wakes up very, very early—like 5am, 6am—and usually is dressed by 7am (so that she's ready for her Dr. K visits around 7:30am). With the time change, that's an easy one for the East Coasters. Morning is a good time for anything that takes energy, including long talks.

Also, it's fine just to sit with her—no need to make conversation. Bring your computer, book, work, whatever. Amy needs her rest and needs to be able to doze off. Constant stimulation/conversation is not necessary.

Make sure Scotty knows that when you're there, you've "got it" so that he is free to do whatever he needs/wants to do. One major benefit of being there for Amy is also freeing up Scott. He's exhausted too, and needs time to do stuff and recharge.

The bungalow has a hair-blower, no need to bring your own.

These are things that just came to mind—some are probably obvious (sorry) but figured I'd share anyway.

Passing the baton of on-the-ground reporter to Jody for current updates. What an amazing network of family and friends Amy and Scotty have.

Jill xo

6

The next afternoon, Lauren arrives just as an IV nurse makes an attempt to slide a new needle into my forearm. My eyes are closed tight, but I can identify my friend's footsteps as she enters the room.

"Lauren!" I open my eyes for just a couple of seconds to take in the happy sight of her.

"Hi, lovey girl," she says, cheerful but terrifically serene. "I see you've got something going on there. Should I step out for a minute?"

I tell her to stay, please; it's just an IV change. With eyes closed again, I hear her settle into the chair beside my bed. She takes my hand in hers.

"Darn it, darn it, ugh . . ." The nurse sighs with exasperation. "I didn't get the vein this time either. Sorry." She places my right arm gently on the bed and takes a deep breath.

It was her third try, and I was verging on tears when Lauren walked in. IVs are harder to insert when the heart is not pumping blood through the veins with requisite strength. The problem is only made worse over time by the daily (or sometimes twice daily) blood draws that inflict innumerable vein punctures, thereby making it even harder to find pristine spots for IV placement. And since IVs have to be removed and relocated every three days to prevent infection, the stretch of available real estate along the arms becomes overpopulated quickly with holes and hematomas. During the two months I spent in the hospital waiting for my first donor heart, I had more than fifty IV changes that became increasingly mangling and agonizing. And now, barely one week into my stay at Cedars, I see my veins moving quickly toward destruction—a portent of many grueling IV changes to come.

"I'm going to give it one more try," the nurse says through a taut smile, "and if it doesn't work this time, I'll get the supervisor, okay?"

"All right." I feel a tear slip through, even though my eyes are shut tight.

Lauren gives my hand a little squeeze. "Okay, honey."

"You're here," I say, just because it comforts me to confirm this out loud.

"I most certainly am."

"Good . . . because . . . *sniff, sniff* . . . it's been so hard, Lauren, and I need . . . I mean, I . . . I'm just so . . . Thank you, thank you . . ." Tears stream down my nose, my cheeks.

"Love you, girl," she says.

"Love you too."

I exhale and settle into the moment.

Everything feels suddenly easier. The unfamiliar hospital room and fraught IV scene that Lauren just walked into do not intimidate her, and I feel at once the power of two in her company. This sense of confident togetherness is something we've earned; it's not a trusted closeness that happened on its own through friendship dating back to childhood, like Jill and I have experienced. Lauren and I didn't meet until we were young adults—and it didn't go too well at first. But our relationship has grown steadily and beautifully since our somewhat shaky beginning.

If you ask Lauren about the first time we met, she will say without hesitation that I wasn't nice to her. "Oh, Amy didn't like me," she'll chide, sort of teasing. Lauren was dating Scott's best friend and law school roommate, Lenny, back then (he's now her husband); getting along as a cozy foursome had been my immediate intent. And yet, as Lauren would tell you, when I answered the doorbell and first laid eyes upon her one Sunday afternoon back in 1987 (Scott and Lenny were in the living room watching football), I hardly offered a warm welcome or introduction. "You said, 'Uh, hi,' and walked immediately into the kitchen," is how Lauren remembers it.

"It wasn't exactly like that."

"Yah-huh, it was."

Whenever Lauren and I revisit this early scene, I try to explain that I'm shy by nature, which happens to be true, but she sees no trace of timidity in me at this point in our long friendship and doesn't buy it. We end up tossing our hands in the air and laughing: We were so young. Who can remember the forces at work when we first met?

I could, actually.

I remember Lauren on that doorstep perfectly. And I have an idea of why I turned away from her at that moment and why still, to this day, I'm taken aback for the first few seconds just about every time I greet her—at the coffee place in town or on the street corner where we start up a neighborhood walk or anywhere, really, even though we're the closest of friends. There's something about Lauren that delays an easy hello.

It's not so much the way she looks, although her attractiveness is striking enough to ignite high-school-level envy and comparisons. Now, at fifty years old, Lauren carries herself effortlessly, with toned muscles and unfailingly perfect posture. But it's not simply physical loveliness that commands Lauren's effect; it's more the way she puts her mind to use and orchestrates success.

I squeeze her hand so tight now, she calls out "Ouch!" right along with me. Even though I've turned my head away from the insertion site, I can feel that the needle isn't in correctly—because it's painful. When an IV is a well-placed keeper, it doesn't hurt much at all.

"Your vein, ugh! Just can't get this in . . ." the nurse laments, removing her gloves and wiping her forehead. "I'm going to get the supervising nurse so I don't have to keep sticking you, sweetheart." She gathers the paraphernalia from atop my blanket—a mess of rubbery tourniquets, paper and plastic discards, used needle sleeves and gauze—and tells me not to worry. "Maybe she'll get lucky and find a good vein—somehow."

Maybe? Somehow? I career my torso up and away from the pillow stack. My mouth flies open to make room for a blast of frustration. Lauren's hand lands on my thigh.

She exhales through her nose and floats at once to standing, as if tied to a helium-filled idea. Taking hold of my left forearm—the one the nurse has not tried yet—Lauren inspects its condition at close range. "Quick question before you go?" she asks amiably, meeting the nurse's eyes directly. "Why not try this arm? I defer to you, of course, but look . . ." She points to a few green-blue veins visible close the surface of my skin.

The nurse tells her that the previous IV had been placed in that arm, and that it's preferable to switch with each change.

Lauren pauses for a second, finger to chin. "Oh, okay, I see. And I respect that, of course. But Amy's had a lot of sticks already—as you so kindly pointed out. Wouldn't it be great to get a sure thing on the next try? Unless you think that having two left-arm IVs in a row would pose a risk to her . . ."

I shift my eyes to the IV nurse—what's her reaction to this layperson suggesting how she might do her job differently?

A slow nod. A kind smile.

Three minutes later, I've got an IV perfectly in place—on the left. If Lauren's solution seemed like an obvious one, it was only because she led us all to it with such ease. In hospital settings, where things are done the same way over and over, whether driven by protocol or mere habit, an agile, genteel approach like hers can save the day. There is a lesson for me in what she has accomplished here—I feel it in the calm that pervades the room in the wake of her grace under pressure. It would do me good to channel it in the days to come. But can I really? Her coolheaded decorum isn't easily emulated, even under the best of circumstances.

As long as I've known Lauren, she's been a thinker. A measured assessor before action. A careful calculator of this moment and the next, and the one after that. When I first met her, I could tell she was confident and prepared, at twenty-three years old, in ways I hadn't given even a moment's consideration. I didn't have the wherewithal to integrate my sense of her into concrete thought just then, but I could gather this much: *This girl has got it together in more ways than I can tell.*

Unlike me at twenty-three years old (or fifty), Lauren was and is completely and consistently in control of her presence. The extent to which she's got her wits about her is instantly apparent and, in my repeated experience, a little daunting. It's not so much jealousy that hits me; it is more a sense of awe at how she lives the cognitive ideal. Careful thought precedes all action. I can't imagine Lauren ever running out of a hospital room and hiding from her friend in a darkened hallway. She'd get a hold of herself.

"Listen to this—I water-skied for the first time in I don't know how many years," she told me just last summer, "and I dropped a ski and did the rest slalom" (on a single ski, that is). "I fell once and told myself, *Lauren, you've got to balance more accurately—pull in that stomach and lean thirty degrees to the left and ten degrees back.* Then I thought about my arms, rotated my left wrist, and brought my right hand into a more dominant position . . ."

I'd gone water-skiing not too long ago as well and, unlike my more analytically gifted friend, gave it no thought: no self-evaluation of my technique, no purposeful adjustment of my position. I just let the boat pull me willy-nilly for a few feet and then belly flopped into the cold lake.

Every time I say hello to my dear friend Lauren, I feel some of that splash.

LEJA IS HOLDING her breath. The tip of her nose has turned red and she's pulled in her chin like a turtle; I'm sure of it, even though I can't see her. We're on the phone. Leja is back in New York for a few days of well-earned rest after spending a month here in California. She blows out a gust of air now and takes in another gulp. This is how Leja weeps.

I'm glad I picked up her call. I had ignored all the other rings and pings from my cell phone over the past few days, but when I saw Leja was calling I told Lauren and Jody I wanted to take it.

"We'll run down for a quick coffee, then," Lauren whispers, giving Jody the nod to join her as I say hello into the cell. I gesture toward the door—*Go ahead . . . I'm fine.*

There is loud sniffling on the other end of the phone. "Leja, breathe," I say gently. "Tell me what's going on."

"I do not want to bother to you. You are in hospital."

"Don't be silly. I'm always here for—"

"Okay, I will tell to you—it's that Brenda! I hear that she is telling to the mothers at the bus stop that I go with my friend to California for fun trip and this is why I quit her house. *For fun trip!*" Leja explains that she's worried this will ruin her reputation and cause trouble when she tries to find another job after returning from California. Beyond the economics of it, she prides herself on being a hardworking and highly trustworthy nanny and house cleaner, and she can't fathom her former boss Brenda speaking ill of her. Leja has made a point of being nothing but discreet and private, never sharing with me anything she sees or hears on the job, never criticizing mothers, fathers, kids, or even unruly dogs in the households where she has worked. And while she has cried to me many times over the last couple of years that she's unhappy working for Brenda (whom I know only as a mere acquaintance), she refrained from saying exactly why; instead, she remained loyal and earnest, wondering aloud to me what she can do to handle the job better and bring a happier attitude to it day after day. She finally decided to return to her affirmations, sitting at the computer for ten-minute concentration sessions once or twice a day, watching her preselected messages trail across the screen: *I enjoy my work . . . I do an excellent job and I feel appreciated . . . Work stresses do not bother me . . .*

When Scott and I asked Leja to consider coming to California with us for an unspecified number of months, she knew this meant ending her job as a nanny and housekeeper for Brenda. And while the prospect of quitting was not an unhappy one for Leja, she was intent on handling it professionally and giving proper notice. Scott and I talked with her about it, and we decided that two weeks was typically fair, figuring that Brenda likely would have given this same duration of additional employ were she to fire Leja.

"Brenda tells to people that I did a bad thing to her family when I decide go to California for fun trip with you. How can she say such!"

Leja had explained to Brenda that she wanted to help me in this terrible time—that I had been a good friend to her, and that in Croatian culture, good friends do all they can for each other without thinking of themselves. But, according to the chatter, Brenda would not believe that Leja's motives did not include California fun. "I felt inside me so terrible when I quit her job. I said to her this, 'Amy is dying' . . . but she kept telling to me, 'Two weeks! How can you leave in two weeks!' I said again to her, 'Amy is dying' . . ."

Leja lets out a squeak of anguish and blows her nose. I've got to assure her that she has done nothing wrong. "Two weeks' notice—that's standard stuff. You shouldn't feel bad about it."

"I feel angry . . . I do a good thing and Brenda says this about me. I do not deserve!"

"No, Leja, you do not deserve it one bit. You are a good person and an excellent worker. You are fair and kind. And you are saving my life." I feel my eyes fill with tears. "Let's talk about it more tomorrow, okay?"

I sit up against some pillows, pull my laptop toward me, and dare to open it. I don't have sufficient strength for emails or even texts; I write almost none these days, and most of the ones I receive go unanswered. But I'm rallying myself to try to set things right for Leja.

Dear Brenda,

I thought of you this morning from my hospital room at Cedars-Sinai, where I'm waiting for a second heart transplant. The biggest help to me as I struggle here is Leja, who is and has long been my Croatian sister, friend, and supporting spirit. It was quite hard for me to ask her to leave her job to help me. But it was quite wonderful that Leja responded to my desperate need with such selflessness, thinking of nothing but how she might help. Just know, for what it's worth, that Leja is doing an angel's work here as I struggle for each breath, hoping for a miracle.

I do hope that things are going great with your family these days . . .

I lift my fingers from the keyboard and fall back against the pillows, exhausted and nauseated. One email is more than my heart's energy allows. I open my night table drawer and reach for my Tums and Tylenol stash—contraband that my friends know I'm harboring against the rules, *naughty, naughty*. No one wants to wait for a nurse to fetch a doctor's written order when they've got nausea or a headache. Secreting away my own Tums and Tylenol is a trick I learned many hospital stays ago, and thank goodness for it: right now I feel close to vomiting. My abdomen has stretched to second-trimester distention, suspiciously firm to the touch and full of the same fluid that has inflated my ankles and feet to near bursting. My liver is now enlarged (due to right-side heart failure, Dr. K tells me), which makes it hard to eat much of anything and inches me toward malnourishment (my blood level of the vital protein albumin is declining, which is a dangerous telltale sign).

The simple breathlessness I felt one month ago when Leja and I spied the auspicious hummingbird in the bungalow garden is but a quaint memory. In the changing of the friend guard from Leja to Jody to Jill to Lauren, my heart problem has become a systemic one. I have come to realize this not just by noting the daily blood results and EKG printouts from my telemetry monitor that the doctors and nurses show me on request. Even more meaningful to me are the watchful measurements I apply to myself each day—little tests I've invented, most of them involving the application of numbers that hark back to my windowpane breath counts. It's a desperate attempt to find my footing in heart failure quicksand.

So, for the last two weeks, I've been counting the duration of my urine flow in seconds. I use this as an indication of my kidney function, which, in turn, gives me insight into whether my heart's failure is causing other organs to fail as well.

Just last night, for instance, I had the urge to pee and got excited that my body would be expelling more of the fluid that now is not only flooding my feet and ankles, but also settling into my lungs in the form of a vapory gurgle. I sat on the toilet, and . . . *one, one thousand . . . two, one thousand . . . three . . .*

Back at the bungalow last month, I made it to ten—which I perceived as something of an unsatisfying dribble at the time. But those days, I realize now, were actually the golden ones, so to speak. My flow time has been on a steady downslide since then: nine, seven, and, at last count, an ominous six—not just at night, but every time I answer the rare urge to pee. And to make it worse, the seven steps I walk from the bathroom back to my hospital bed (and yes, of course, I count them) bring on a spate of heartbeat fireworks in my chest that linger long after I've lain back down again. I don't even try to count and assess these beats because I know I can't. The disappearing pulse that sent me to Cedars's ER is a permanent fixture now; the pumping of my heart has become so feeble, it is imperceptible at all pulse points.

Leja picked up on this new sign of heart failure just a few days ago. "You feel now it is much more weak, your heart?" she asked, watching my fingers fly from my wrist to the top of my foot and then to a spot directly over my heart—all places where I might land on a beating sensation.

My hands flew again—this time to cover my face as I answered her. "I don't know, I don't know . . . I can't feel my heartbeat anymore. Not anywhere . . ." My voice dropped to a breathy whisper. "And Leja—*it makes me think I'm dead!*"

"Oh, my friend!" She sprang from her chair, lunging toward me with outstretched arms.

Yeah, sure, Brenda—we've been having terrific fun out here in California.
More like one friend disappearing before the other one's eyes.
Your disease is galloping along . . .
A few words from Dr. K could set Brenda straight . . .

I chew on a couple of Tums while looking over my email. "Too neutral," I say out loud to no one. Sure, I'm tugging at Brenda's conscience by detailing Leja's lifesaving presence here in California; speaking ill of an angel is bad form. There's some chance that I can lift Brenda's goodness by exalting Leja's, after all. But my words, as I reread them, seem too mild in response to the bus-stop gossip that is causing my sweet friend to weep.

I need to add some kick to this email. Seeing my words through Leja's eyes, I feel the lack in them; laying guilt and hoping for a shift in Brenda's behavior does not show sufficient fight on behalf of my friend. Leja would be gloves-off and swinging wildly without a second thought if my reputation were attacked—I'm sure of it. Our loyalty toward each other has never been lighthearted. Weakened as I am, I've got to make my words strong for Leja's defense. My first impulse is to ease her angst—always.

I push my fists into the mattress below me and straighten up to a sitting position. With fingers on the keyboard now, I clench my molars with determination—*Come on, Amy, add some bite to this thing . . .*

A few minutes later, Lauren and Jody walk in holding giant Starbucks cups. "And she wants red . . ." Lauren says. They're talking prom dresses; it's mid-March and high school senior girls are already posting their dresses on Facebook and, thereby, *claiming* them. Lauren brings me into the conversation. "Red isn't a popular color, so Carly's probably safe in waiting a few weeks to choose hers."

"Mmm, red. Bold," I say.

Jody starts to lower herself into the chair nearest to the door, and Lauren gets ruffled. "Uh, mind if I take that one, Jo? I've, uh, got all my stuff next to it . . ." Jody's eyes pop as she lets out an *ah, right!* sound that seems to say, *Thanks for reminding me!*

Hmmm.

It would be no surprise if they conferred about ideal chair position-ing outside my earshot (Jody and Lauren are longtime friends, having lived in the same small New York City apartment building when their kids were babies). Whatever they might have worked out, Lauren has sat to the left of my bed and Jody to the right every day so far. But I didn't realize there might be a purpose behind it until just this minute.

I reflect now on how Lauren has been up and down from that chair and back and forth from the door many times over the last few days. It seems she has been standing guard, managing all admittance to my room since she got here. I hadn't given it a second thought, but now I have an idea of why Lachalle hasn't been in for the two a.m. blood pressure check for the last couple of nights. The schedule for nurse's aides is strict on the cardiac floor: ten p.m., two a.m., six a.m. But after Lauren's first night sleeping in my room—and the frequent pacemaker firings had her flying from her bed to mine many times—Lachalle's middle-of-the-night visits dropped off.

"Hey, Lauren, have you noticed—no blood pressure check the last couple of nights?" I ask, interrupting the prom discussion, which has now moved onto danceable shoes. "Lachalle has been leaving me alone."

"Yup, that's right. I spoke with Dr. Lunchbox about it. I told him you're up all night with pacemaker pain and it makes no sense to wake you *again* for a silly blood pressure check when what you really need is rest. He wrote an order that's been posted outside your door every night, saying you're not to be woken 'til six."

So *that's* what she was talking with Dr. Lunchbox about in the hall-way the other day. And it dawns on me that I haven't had to gather myself to chat with the heart transplant volunteers—mostly older men who pull down the necks of their T-shirts to show me their sternum scars ("Can hardly see it, right?") while waxing enthusiastic about how great my life will be with a donor heart—or the hospital representatives who check in room by room to see if patients are comfortable, or the always-cheerful housekeeping supply replenisher, or the day's supervising nurse who just wants to introduce herself and say hi. Within twenty-four hours of arriving here, Lauren assessed what might make my days and nights a little less taxing, and she set to it. She'd also had Jill's emails to go on, and it seems Jill passed the baton to Lauren in a way that would help her to hit the ground running when she arrived.

And then, as I would expect, Lauren added to it her methodical maneuvering. Poor Dr. Lunchbox—he didn't stand a chance when Lauren cornered him in the hallway with a firm request. No doubt she stood a full head taller than this newbie cardiac resident and held immediate sway over him with her poise. I'm sure her hallway recitation showed careful forethought: she would be respectful of the doctor's time and would say so right up front, and then she likely dazzled with specifics: *Amy is up during the night an average of five times, with pacing pain lasting approximately fourteen minutes each go-round, which means seventy minutes of wakened, painful state and about one hundred ten minutes left for sleep between blood pressure, uh . . . What is it, Dr. Baird?* (He'd be looking a little dumbfounded by now.) *You're wondering if I've been taking notes for the last three nights? Yes. What do you say the nurse's aide skips the two a.m.?*

Done.

"Wow, thanks so much for that," I say to Lauren. "I've spent a lot of nights in the hospital but never thought to ask for a *Do Not Disturb* sign on my door."

"Well, there was no way around it. I had to speak up," Lauren replies. "You need your sleep."

And Leja needs to preserve her reputation. Small-town gossip spreads exponentially and sticks. I flip open my computer and press send on my punched-up email to Brenda.

Jody rises to gather her things, telling Lauren how great it was to spend these past few mornings together. "Wish it were under different circumstances, but ya know, when do I get to sit with two New York friends and talk for hours?" she says. They link arms and walk to the elevator. When Lauren returns, she resumes her watchful post in the chair near the door—straight spine, lifted chin.

"You're sitting there on purpose, aren't you?" I say.

"Sure am. You don't need people bothering you all day. I only let in the important ones. I want to do my best for you every minute I'm here."

"Sounds exhausting."

"To you, maybe. Not to me. I have only four days in this hospital room, and then I go back to my regular life. Sure, things are going to be pretty chaotic when I return tomorrow night, but I'm going to get into my bed and sleep 'til morning. I'll be restored in no time."

"But you didn't sign on for *this*. The spreadsheet visits were supposed to be different. We all thought I'd spend my waiting list days at the bungalow, not in a hospital room. We were going to hang out in the little garden, enjoy the sun . . ."

Lauren leans in and looks into my eyes. "Amy, I never thought that," she says, clear and solemn. "I don't think any of the girls did."

"Then how could all of you commit to this in the first place? How could that spreadsheet fill up so fast?"

"I can't speak for anyone else. But for me, it wasn't even a question. I would've been disappointed in myself if I didn't come to California— I'd be letting you *and* myself down."

"You wouldn't be letting me down. I would understand."

There's a long pause. Lauren is devising a thoughtful response. She pushes her hair behind her ears and stares off for a moment, moving her lips a little as if reciting a grocery list to herself before entering the supermarket. "Okay, now I'm going to sound selfish," she finally says. "But here's what you need to know. I love you—well, you know that— and I feel that you and I have a special place in each other's lives. We're logical thinkers, we walk each other through the big hard things step by step and figure them out together. You hear me and understand me, and I've tried so hard to do the same for you. And you know . . . here comes the selfish part . . . I feel I've done a really good job at that. I'm your consigliere, right, and this makes me feel good about myself, like it's validating that you've chosen me. I think I have a lot to offer."

I make a fist and bring it to my lips. I want to absorb these words, remember them. The honesty of this moment whirs toward me—bright, forceful, nearly blinding. *This is once-in-a-lifetime, Amy. Open your eyes.*

Lauren continues without pause: "My friendship with you, it's a source of pride because I've come through for you, Amy—my best self every time. So if you ask what I'm doing here, well, I'm doing what I've always done and what I've really wanted to do—only this time, it's in a different location."

My mouth slackens in surprise. I've always thought that my being sick is nothing but a drain on my friends. Leave it to Lauren to articulate a completely different perspective.

In this moment, I'm a mirror of Lauren's emotions. Pride, validation, and love are pulsing through me. Lauren has chosen our friendship to be a measure of herself—how can I not feel energized to bring my best self to it, even during this most trying time?

"Feel better now, silly? Call me selfish, but I'm glad I said all this," she says.

I do feel better. But I think the words she just shared with me may be the most selfless I've ever heard.

LATER THAT DAY, motion by the door sends Lauren charging toward it, but just after reaching the entryway vestibule she retreats with an apology.

"No worries," I hear someone say to her, and then Dr. Kobashigawa enters the room. "Afternoon, afternoon!" he pipes.

There it is again, his double greeting: the time of day recited twice in quick succession (Dr. K's double time, as I've come to call it). His cadence is always upbeat, at least at first. "Oh, Scott, hello. I'm glad you're here," he says.

Scott comes early every morning to see Dr. K during rounds, but he varies his afternoon hours here with me. Leja, Jill, and now Lauren try consistently to push him out of the room, saying, "Take some time for yourself, please, Scotty. We're here with Amy so that you don't have to be." They urge him to get some air, go for a run, or take a shower for crying out loud. Part of the objective of the spreadsheet is to help *him*, they say. But Scott rebuffs their orders night and day. He will slide onto my hospital bed at night, preferring to nod off beside me for an hour or so, squished, rather than sleep comfortably in his bed a just few blocks away. Then he'll slide back in again at daybreak for an hour or so—first handing off a Starbucks Grande to the visiting guest—before rushing back to the bungalow for the first business call of the day.

Lauren was just about to kick him out this afternoon when Dr. K arrived. She offers the doctor her chair.

"All right," he says, leaning onto his forearms and clasping his hands. "I have something to talk to you about . . ."

Hope flashes across Lauren's face—*Maybe he's got news about a new heart!* But I know this can't be it; a donor heart match needs no introductory words. I'm also familiar enough at this point with Dr. K's style to know when he's couching something unpleasant.

"Now. Have you heard of a total artificial heart?"

"Yeah, I know about it. But if you're thinking I would agree to one of those . . ."

"I'm not saying *now*. But the approach of our team here at Cedars is to stay one step ahead. We don't want things to nosedive suddenly and force us—and you—to make decisions under pressure. Let's line things up so we're ready to move if we have to."

"What aren't you telling me?" My voice is louder than I want it right now, and more intense. I always try to hang on to calm when speaking with Dr. Kobashigawa; I don't want to lose his respect before I've known him long enough to secure it. But this moment is harking straight back to Columbia, where, for twenty-five touch-and-go transplant years, my doctor fed me bad news one encrypted bread crumb at a time until I found myself under a deathly heap, suffocating. *Cedars isn't Columbia—use your mind, choose your words carefully,* I remind myself, trying to pattern after Lauren's displays of self-control. *Dr. Kobashigawa has been nothing but straight with you.* I try again. "I mean, what's the chance that I might need an artificial heart?"

"I don't know. But I will say—and I'm sure this comes as no surprise—your condition is deteriorating more rapidly than expected. You heart failure is now biventricular, which means it's on both the right and left sides . . ." The right side of my heart is supposed to pump blood to my lungs—that's where it gets oxygen. Then the left side takes that blood and pumps it through my body to my other organs— kidneys, liver, brain.

"So neither side is doing the job it needs to do," I reply.

"Yes, exactly right," Dr. Kobashigawa says, "and this is the cardiogenic shock I talked about last week. Your heart is becoming less and less responsive to the pacemaker. I see it on the telemetry reports. At some point the pacemaker won't work at all."

"And that's when I'll die."

Scott shoots me a look—*Stop being provocative.*

"Ah, *heh-heh,* Amy, somehow I knew you'd say that. I'm getting to know you better by the day," Dr. Kobashigawa says, smiling with his eyes for a few seconds before turning serious again. "Now. With the total artificial heart, what would happen is—"

"I don't need to hear it."

"Well, I do," Scott says. He's annoyed with me now. "Please go on."

I look out the window while the doctor explains to Scott what I already know about this "bridge to transplant," as it's called. A total artificial heart is not a permanent alternative to a transplanted heart, but rather a temporary pumping device placed inside the chest cavity until a matching donor heart becomes available.

"We would remove Amy's current heart entirely and replace it with . . ."

I look over at Lauren. She's taking notes. I turn my head back toward the window.

"It's not without risk—and inconvenience. It's open-heart surgery, of course, a full opening of the sternum. Amy would have to remain in the hospital here for six months of recovery after this surgery, during which time she would be taken off the transplant waiting list. After that, she would be back on the list and start the wait again."

Scott shakes his head. "Six months of recovery from open-heart, and *then* get on the transplant waiting list?" His reaction matches mine, thank goodness. Scott is remembering the horrible months of recovery following my valve surgery just a year or so ago. I have to assume he's also made a quick calculation of how long our California stay could last in the wake of this surgery and my being relisted for heart transplant: a year, or maybe more.

"Yes. But it could save her life . . . *your* life, Amy." I feel the doctor's gaze upon me and turn to meet it now. "We have great success with artificial hearts here. There's a young man on the other side of this building who's got one right now—I'm sure he'd be happy to come talk with you about it."

"Mmm, thank you, but no. I'm not going to do an artificial heart." Lauren stops scribbling and stares at me. Scott looks down at the ground, unable to mask his sadness. But I go on. "You're getting to know me a little, Dr. Kobashigawa, but what you don't realize is that, for me, death is an option—a real choice that I see as totally legitimate and rational. I'm not twenty-five this time around. I've raised my son. I've had incredible years with Scott, all of them bonus years, as I see it. And I've given this donor heart every last ounce of my energy and devotion—kept it beating for way, way longer than any doctor expected.

But now it might just be my time to die. We all die. I'm just going to die sooner than everyone I know."

He tugs one side of his white coat over the other and chuckles a little. "Ah, Amy, that's not very optimistic . . ."

"With all due respect—and there's a lot due here, that I know—you're the one asking me to look at the worst-case scenario. I'm just saying that I will choose—that I *am* choosing, and firmly—not to do a total artificial heart. And I think . . . well, I *hope* . . . that Scott will support my choice. And meanwhile—here's some optimism for you—*let's get me a donor heart before I croak.*" I'm feeling lighter by the minute, content that I've spoken my mind, and appreciative that Dr. K gave me the time and space to do so. It's not a happy choice, sure, but there's tremendous relief in finally being able to say no to exponential suffering.

Dr. Kobashigawa stands up and shakes Scott's hand and Lauren's, and then, more slowly and with steady eye contact, mine. "Think about it, all right?"

I smile, closemouthed. "Mmm."

Scott follows him into the hall.

Lauren closes her wire-bound notebook and looks up at me. "We'll talk about this?" she asks.

"Yeah. But you can't be surprised at my decision."

"I'm not. It's a big one, though. It's got real consequences. You've got to be completely sure . . ."

Scott walks in looking dazed.

"Why don't you go back to the bungalow for a little while and get some rest. I've got it covered here," Lauren says to him.

Before he leaves, though, I want to make sure we're together on this. "Open-heart surgery, Scotty. Six months in the hospital. *Then* the waiting list. It could be a year or more in California. What about your work? And for me, what about all the . . . I mean, you know there's going be trauma and horror with that artificial heart. I don't have room in my brain for any more of it . . . I just don't!" My voice cracks and my eyes brim with tears.

Scott climbs on my bed and lies down beside me. We contort immediately into our usual body-braid tangle—legs over legs, feet against feet, arms entwined with arms, head tipped against head. "It's awful. It's horrific," he says, "and . . . I won't ask you to do it for *me*." I feel his teardrops on my neck.

"Good. Because I can't, I can't do it, Scotty. It's beyond me. We'll just have to wait for a heart and hope I make it."

"Yeah." He sits up and wipes the base of his palm across his eyes. Lauren wipes her own eyes with a tissue. We all sit quietly together for a minute. There's no sense of embarrassment among us. No awkwardness. Lauren has long been a close friend of both of ours, and she's not simply a witness here; rather, she is, in the truest way, a full part of this excruciating and profound moment in my life, in my marriage, and, more than likely, in my death; everything is intense and open and extraordinarily real. The world stops spinning for a minute—a minute that's soul-sinking and awful, but also somehow transcendent and valuable.

No one said the unadorned essence of life and death is pretty. It sure is something to behold, though.

Scott gives me a kiss and gets up from the bed. "Okay, I'll go rest a little," he says. "I'll bring some dinner for all of us later."

LAUREN READS FROM her notebook. "Dr. Kobashigawa says the surgery would be about seven hours. Well, you've done longer ones."

"The valve surgery," I say. "It was a nightmare."

"And then six months recovery—in the hospital, he says—"

"No way."

"And then you get back on the waiting list."

"But with an even higher number of antibodies. Did you hear him say that?" Dr. Kobashigawa explained that my body would consider the total artificial heart itself to be foreign, and that this would cause increased antibody production—a sort of rejection phenomenon. "Right now I'm able to take a donor heart from only about fourteen percent of the population because of my ridiculously high antibodies. With the artificial heart inside me, I'd have an even worse chance for a donor match."

"He did say that, yes. But he also said that donor matches have been found for patients who could only accept hearts from one percent of the population, and that means—"

"Can we stop this?"

She drops her chin and peers at me over her reading glasses. "Of course." The notebook closes in her lap. "We can talk later. You don't have to make a decision on this right away."

"Lauren, I've already made my decision."

"Ah . . . but . . ."

"I need you to be on my side." I begin to tremble.

"It's not about sides. We're talking this through, taking it apart like we always do . . ."

My brain goes fuzzy with anger. "You want me to get this ridiculous contraption in my chest—cut my heart out and put a friggin' motor in there and then rot in the hospital for six months?"

"No. I didn't say that."

"You're pushing me to do what's good for *you*, not for *me*!" My hands ball into fists at my side. The situation strikes an explosive chord in me. There's something about the casual tone of Lauren's voice—insistence cloaked in a *let's wait and see* timbre—that suggests I'm being irrational and need careful stringing along until I come to my senses. I've heard this affected nonchalance before, but this time I can't keep myself from challenging it directly. Frustration grabs me by the throat now. Words come flying from my mouth. "This is just like what happened that day with the police. I still haven't forgiven you for that."

Lauren looks away. She's biting her lower lip. I've brought up a terribly sore spot between us—something we've never talked about, but rather let fall away from us, unexplained. It is an awful memory, still raw, of an upheaval that rocked our relationship.

The ordeal occurred just three months before the bad-news an-
giogram (and four months before I headed out to California): a breast
sonogram picked up a strange-looking spot in my right breast. I didn't
worry at first because soon after my first transplant, the regimen of
immunosuppressive medicines caused benign fibroadenoma masses
to grow in my breasts. They were easily spotted on sonograms and
sometimes grew so large I had to get them surgically removed. But this
particular spot looked different. When I asked the biopsy radiologist if
she thought she'd just put a needle into something scary, she threw up
her hands. "Gosh, this is a weird-looking one," she said. "I don't know
what it is."

It was cancer.

Of all the emotions and questions that followed, *Why me?* was not
among them. Transplant medicines are strongly linked to cancers, es-
pecially after imposing decades of immunosuppressive wrath on the
body. Added to this menace were the seventy-nine heart biopsies and
twenty-eight angiograms I'd had—all of them done under powerful X-
rays to the chest with no localized protection since the heart area was
being imaged. I was a breast cancer lump waiting to happen. And so
it did.

When I got the post-biopsy call from my breast doctor, Scott hap-
pened to be on his way to Las Vegas with Lenny and another friend
to meet Jack for a weekend of golf. They'd planned this trip for a long
time, and I insisted that he go, even though I was waiting on a test
result. The moment he landed, my doctor called him with the news—
even before she spoke with me (a break from usual protocol, but this
doctor had been my transplant physician since the beginning). Scott
and his friends never left the airport; they retrieved their bags and got
on the next flight back to New York.

When she reached me with the news, I froze.

"Oh, come on! With all you've been through, this is easy stuff!"
my breast doctor implored. She couldn't have chosen more enraging
words. I'd known this doctor since I started growing those golf ball

fibroadenomas just after my first transplant, and I liked her a lot. But she was barking up a dangerous tree at a tragic moment by trying to turn my years of illness into a rallying call, when I was seeing it as a signal to raise the white flag.

"I'm not doing it," I said. "I had a horrid open-heart valve surgery just a few months ago. And, frankly, my heart isn't feeling so great lately. I'm not taking on breast cancer. I'm . . . I'm out."

Ooh. Nice.

I liked the feel of these words as they rolled off my lips for the first time—*I'm out*.

"You can't quit now! You have to fight this. You're just the kind of person who's going to do great—"

"I'm out! I'm out! I'm out!" Wow, I loved the sound—and the sentiment. *I'm free! I don't have to do this anymore!* For me, taking on an additional life-threatening illness was completely unfathomable. It was so beyond okay or understandable or doable or fair. "I gotta go now . . ."

"Go where?"

And this is where I made a really big mistake. "I'm leaving," I said. "I'm getting in the car now. I'm not doing this anymore."

"You can't. You have to do this. Amy! Let's talk! Would you come to the city and meet with me? I'll cancel my afternoon . . ."

"Bye."

I left.

And then I was driving, blindly. My cell phone rang and it was Scott, telling me that my breast doctor called the local police because she's worried about me. The police were at the house now, he said, and Lauren was on the way to meet them. He told me to go back home. "I'm out!" I cried, and kept driving.

I didn't know where I was headed, but the distance from my house took on urgency now; this was an escape. The speedometer shot from fifty-five to seventy. I switched on the radio, found a hard rock station, and turned the volume way up. I opened the windows and let the ice-cold air inflate my anger. No way I was turning around. There was a party going on at my house, for fuck's sake, with law enforcement and everything.

Lauren moves now from her watch post by the door to the chair nearest my bed. She's got tears in her eyes, but her mouth is set with determination. "You say you haven't forgiven me for that day. Well, you don't know what really happened with the police. I haven't told you because things moved so quickly from the breast stuff to your needing a second transplant—I didn't feel it was important to explain myself. Until now."

The hospital room seems to shrink around us. The moment narrows and we teeter on its edge. Our eyes lock as Lauren begins to tell the story I do not know.

"I get a call from Lenny and he says to go to your house because the police are coming. I don't know if you're there or not, but I race over," she explains. "I pull up to your house and there are three cop cars and they are *on your lawn*—why they didn't park on the driveway, I don't know. I go to your door, and the police have busted through the window. I walk in and hear them in your bedroom, so I head upstairs and they're rifling through your closet and drawers—clothes are everywhere. One of them has got your journal and he's standing there reading it. I think to myself, *I have a job to do. I have to protect Amy.* And I dive into conversation with those cops, rambling on and on, pretending to be helpful. They ask me what color your car is, and I waste ten minutes saying, *Hmmm, I don't know.* They ask if you were likely to head north or south, I tell them north—because I know you're much more likely to go south . . ."

I get a call from Lauren, and I don't pick up. Another call, and I don't pick up.

"I keep trying your cell, but you won't answer. The cops are asking me, 'Would she hurt herself?' and I tell them no. She got some really bad news and she wants to be alone. I know her well. She's fine. But they tell me I have to call you again because they want you back here. They put an alert out on your car."

Meanwhile, I call my breast doctor and the receptionist puts me right through. "Why did you call the police!" I shout. "It's my choice to fight breast cancer or not. You've known me so many years, you've seen all I've been through—how can you force a decision on me? I can't believe you did this!"

"I'm sorry, I'm sorry. I'll call them back. It just sounded like you might do something . . ."

"I'm fine. I'm upset because . . . how many times and in how many ways can I be dying? I'm not going to drive off a bridge, for God's sake! And even if I did, that would be my business." I'm shuddering with anger.

"But I'm under legal obligation, Amy. I could get in trouble if I know you are going to hurt yourself and then you do."

"Well, I'm not going to hurt myself. But I am not going to take on breast cancer either. I just had valve surgery. It's my choice."

"I'll call the police and tell them everything is okay, but you have to come and meet me to talk. I'll meet you at my house or at Starbucks near my office if you want. I just want to lay out what the treatment would be so you can make an informed choice."

"Okay, I'll meet you. Four thirty. Starbucks. Now call the police and tell them I'm fine!"

A few seconds later, Lauren calls again, and this time I pick up. She asks me if I'm all right.

"I need time alone. I don't need another person telling me I have to fight breast cancer, blah blah blah!" I tear at the zipper on my winter coat, tugging it down as I shake my shoulders out from underneath, frenzied. I am boiling with fury.

She tells me the police are there. My doctor hasn't reached them yet.

"I heard. And I know everyone wants me to come home and be a good

little breast cancer–valve surgery–heart transplant patient, just racking up
the life-threatening illnesses and their shitty, half-assed treatments—"

"Yes . . ." is her reply, and it's like a quick slap in the face. It's as if what I
want has no value. It's as if I have no agency.

I burst out at her, "I have to say, Lauren, after all we've talked about all
these years, and with all that you know about me and the unbelievable shit
I've had to endure to stay alive since I was twenty-five fucking years old,
I would expect you'd be more understanding. But no. You're not on my
side!"

I am battled out. How can she not see this?

"Mmm-hmm . . ." she says. There's noise in the background. I can hear a
police officer saying something about a call from my doctor. "Oh, so you're
meeting your doctor at Starbucks in half an hour. That's good. The police
chief says you should have your doctor call him when you're with her, and
then they'll get out of here."

Lauren takes a tissue box from the windowsill now, pulls one out
and then offers me the box. "So while I'm waiting to reach you on the
phone, I call the window-repair place in town and I ask them to come
right away, but it was late in the day on a Friday. The guy says he'll come
after the weekend, but I beg him, please, my friend is ill. I didn't want
you to come home and see the huge mess of glass all over the place. I
swept that up," she tells me softly. "Vacuumed too . . ."

She also folded and put away all the clothes that the police had
dumped onto the floor from my drawers. And the minute the police
chief was done inspecting my journals, she placed them back in my
night table drawer. "Then, finally, you pick up my call, thank God.
And here's what you need to understand—I was trying to think and
plan ahead the whole time, to figure out what was best for you. When
I called you, I knew I needed to position myself across the room from
where all the cops were standing. But they don't want me way over

there because they want to hear everything you're saying to me. So I tell them, 'If you want her to open up, you'd better keep the walkie-talkies away from me,' and I plant myself on the couch. Then you get on the phone and start asking me if I'm on your side, and what am I supposed to do? The cops are watching me, they're listening to my responses. I can't say, *I support any choice you make*, because I'm trying like hell to protect you."

She pauses and takes a breath. "It was one of the hardest moments in my life—I had to act calm and neutral when I was completely overwhelmed and under pressure. And then you're yelling at me, saying I'm the worst friend."

"I had no idea . . ."

"I know, and that's okay, I understand why you thought I was being awful to you. But I hope you realize now—I was trying to be the best friend I could to you in that moment. And all these months, you didn't know."

We hadn't spoken about it since then. Lauren was in my kitchen when I got home—and so were Jill and another friend, Jane. I went up to my room, and they stayed put until Scott arrived a couple of hours later. Less than a week after that, I underwent a double mastectomy. But I never for a minute saw the undertaking as a courageous, life-saving fight on my part. It was more a giving in—a ceding to what seemed like the normal, rational thing for a woman of my age to do. I was not afraid of major surgery (I'd had my sternum severed by a chain saw more than once, after all). I was not one to grieve the loss of my breasts (parting with my natural-born heart at twenty-five felt far more devastating).

And, if only to escape friends and family urging me to "just think about it . . . just think about it," I did the opposite and dove right into a commitment to mastectomy the day after the police left my house. It felt to me so much easier to just walk the walk of saving my life than talk the talk of what I really felt—which was that my heart wasn't going to last too much longer anyway, so why bother? I had been feeling burning cardiac pain down my arms by then—felt it spread into my neck and chin too when I walked the hundred yards from the breast biopsy suite to my car. But I didn't tell anyone.

Turns out there were a lot of things about that time that we all kept to ourselves.

"I'm incredibly"—*breath*—"sorry, Lauren," I tell her, feeling my lungs weighed down by the details she has just given me.

"*I'm* sorry that I made you think I wasn't on your side," she says, furrowing her brow. "And you've got to know now—with this total artificial heart . . . I support your choices. Maybe I wouldn't have felt the same way ten years ago, but I've seen you suffer terribly over the last few years, and in my mind, the breast cancer was the last straw. The last valiant effort required of you. But then there was more in store for you—who would have thought that a couple months later, you'd be in California on a waiting list for retransplant. Amy, I believe you can do any physical feat, but it's gotten to the point where enough is enough."

She gets it. I feel a rush of gratitude—and remorse.

"I am so sorry I said those things to you on the phone . . ."

"Yeah, well, it was hard to take. I went home and cried about it—a lot. Because there I was, doing all I could for you, and I was proud and grateful to be the one who *could* do it. The whole time it was happening, I kept thinking, *I'm so glad* I'm *the one who's here first. I can give Amy what she needs—some space to process this really bad news.*" Jill and Jane were on their way to the house as well, she tells me, but by the time they got there, I'd already made it to Starbucks to talk to my doctor.

"Honestly, I wasn't really *processing* the bad news," I admit to her now. "I was acting on it. But not in the way everyone thought. I didn't get into my car that day to kill myself—because I didn't have to. My body has been plenty good at dying without any help from me, and then, voilà, look at that, there's breast cancer to speed things along. I was just so ready to say *I'm out* at that point—death by *omission*, if you know what I mean."

Lauren nods. "I do."

"And so, now, saying no to the artificial heart is—"

"I understand," she says, and I believe her.

THE FIRST HINT of sun grazes the windowsill, and I wake to the clickity-squeak of metal wheels approaching my door. Lauren jumps from her cot and bolts to the entryway like a mother to a crying newborn, all instinct and protective drive. "No, no . . . not today," she whispers, and I hear the wheels retreat into the hallway. Lauren has just spared me this morning's weigh-in. She shuffles back to bed, gets under the covers, and settles in for a little more sleep. In two hours, she will head to the airport.

"I don't want to leave you," she said last night, a few minutes after coaching me through a particularly rough pacemaker firing.

"Yeah," was all I could get out before emotion grabbed my throat.

"We did good, though," she added, sitting herself down beside me on the bed and taking my hands in hers. "We work well together."

She's right. During Lauren's four-day visit, she finagled a few helpful changes—from the nighttime *Go Away* sign on my door to the easing up on daily weigh-ins and hourly urine measures. We'd also come up with a sleep plan, as she called it (a euphemism, because the increasing number of pacemaker episodes kept us both up most of the night). According to the plan, at ten o'clock we are each to be in our separate beds. I am to watch some mindless show downloaded to my laptop (*Scandal*, in honor of Joy) and then go to sleep. No talking allowed, just quiet calm. I am supposed to wake Lauren the minute I feel pain; she'll sit on my hospital bed and try to soothe me with light fingernail strokes up and down my back. And then it's bonus time: a test we've come up with to help move me through the duration of pacing. Without looking at the heart monitor screen, we see if I can pinpoint the precise moment when the pacemaker stops firing—this way, we can look forward to relief in just a minute or so.

"And . . . *now!*" is how I call it out, marking the instant at which I feel my heartbeat climb above eighty. Lauren watches the monitor:

she's learned not only how to identify the pulse number in blue, but also how to read the particular line of the EKG that spikes exaggeratedly when my heart is pacing—and she tells me if I am correct.

"You got it! Exactly to the second. It's amazing how well you know your body!"

"It's easy to feel, actually. My heart's inside my chest, you know. Just underneath some skin and bone."

"Give yourself some credit, would you? The way you breathe through that awful pain is incredibly brave. It's like labor, only you have it every night and you're not cursing at your husband," she says with a laugh. "And then you manage somehow to feel *exactly* when your pulse starts to go up. I'm in awe."

"Stop it."

"I will not. What you do is incredible."

I pause, savoring her words. "I have to say, no one ever tells me that. Thank you, Lauren, really, thank you." Her compliment is a rare but welcome affirmation.

"Well then, I'm just going to have to hang around you more so you can hear it more often."

But Lauren is leaving shortly for New York.

Shaking off all signs of sleep deprivation, she'll slip on her black suede booties that haven't come out from under the cot since she got here and wheel her little carry-on through that airport. She will be sure to email the girls while waiting to board the plane, following a protocol of group communication forged by Jill—a protocol that is as much for my benefit as it is for the next friend whose name appears on the spreadsheet. Lauren's ability to implement helpful adjustments within hours of arriving in my hospital room may be thanks, in part, to Jill's detailed reports and suggestions. But the goal Lauren set for herself was her own: "I want to do my very best for you every minute I'm here," she said.

And she's done this in the form and style I would expect—so smooth around the sharp turns of these days and nights at my side, steering through the specter of a total artificial heart, gearing up for cyclical agony, and heading straight into the truth about the day I called her a terrible friend. Lauren has glided along the landscape seamlessly.

Yes, it sometimes is hard to say hello to my friend Lauren. But once you ride with her for a little while, it's much, much harder to say good-bye.

I thought God would protect me. Maybe it would be Jesus doing the work, I don't know. I was born to Jewish parents and raised completely without religion, but we had a housekeeper for a while when I was very young, and she taught me that God is everywhere, which only made me feel bad at first because it meant that every time I sat down, I was crushing him with my butt cheeks. "No, he can't be under there," Ena instructed. "Always above you! That's where God is." I think I was helping her sort socks at the time—a task that made me proud at six years old—and I laid my little body out on the cold basement floor and looked up at the lattice of wooden rafters and steel beams.

"Ena," I whispered, pointing at a single crisscross, "there!"

She fanned herself with a creased, dusty brown hand while her eyes fluttered toward the ceiling. "Jesus! Lord Jesus, amen!" He was hovering, I guess.

Still, it took a while until I felt right about sitting down.

I had a sense of something grand and protective up there or out there— perhaps bearded, perhaps in cloud form, or light or fire—and I carried this sense with me long after Ena returned home to her daughters in Costa Rica. She scratched out letters to me every so often, one of the last coming on the thinnest airmail paper imaginable. "I'm ninety-seven now," she wrote. "God is calling me." I wrote back and told her that he seemed to be calling me too, even though I was only twenty-five. She answered one final time before leaving this world and me. "He holds you in his hand, child."

Then a donor match came through and I was blessed with a healthy heart again. Scott and I got married. Casey arrived and I became a mother. Feeling safe and saved, I had to explain God to myself anew, and it seemed only right to do it this way: God—whoever and whatever that may be—couldn't stop my heart from failing, not for lack of powerfulness, but because, well, it's not possible to watch every little thing all the time; some bad stuff falls through the cracks. But he sure stepped in and made certain that I lived. My being alive was not mere coincidence; heart transplants had just become successful right around 1988. If my heart had failed a few years earlier, say, when I was eighteen instead of twenty-four, I would have died. It's reasonable to say that God held me up until science caught up to my heart's disease. And he sent Scott to me—just in time. And then Casey too, right at the point when I could receive him.

God—or fate or karma or the pull of the universe—may not always have omnipresent vision, but with focus, he-she-it can be very good indeed. How could I not feel the proof of this? Of something making things right after they went so wrong for me? Of a force that recognized that I'd climbed the tall, terrible mountain towering in front of me and was carrying a heavy burden still, which ensured protection from further onslaughts of enormous ill fate?

Breast cancer?

Nah. Not possible. Not me. That's for other women—the ones who haven't had to lose their natural-born hearts.

Lightning can't strike twice. God–fate–karma–the universe wouldn't allow it.

It's the same reasoning I've given to family members and friends who've admitted to being afraid as we've boarded airplanes together. I've got a great way to calm them. "Relax," I say. "I am not a likely person to die on a plane. It would be against the order of all things in the cosmos. Just too darn incongruous. So long as you're flying with me, you should figure you're safe."

But then: breast cancer.

Uh, God?

7

The third pacemaker firing of the night—an especially lengthy one—ended about an hour ago, returning Joy at long last to her cot, exhausted. But I'm still up. Watching the EKG monitor. Considering whether to reach for my cell phone on the night table beside me so I can read some of the texts and emails that have been piling up. Maybe even try to answer one or two.

Nope. Can't do it.

Can't even imagine doing it, really.

My apathy worries me because I sense that it is tied to a deeper message of warning from my body. A lack of desire to do simple acts—especially those that were once habitual or pleasant—is my heart's way of keeping me from expending even the smallest bit of energy, because no act of movement is safe anymore. Each blood-pumping heartbeat is now a blessed bonus, not a casual occurrence to be relied upon. I can feel it. My heart reminds me again and again that I must manage it—very, very carefully.

I know this because I experienced the same phenomenon a couple of years ago, after my valve surgery. At the time I wondered what might be behind my reluctance to do the simplest, most ordinary things (even after my surgical incision had healed), because I was determined to rise above whatever it was. And when, finally, I forced myself to move around freely, refusing to treat my heart like a baby in need of constant tending, I wound up in a fit of palpitations that had me dialing 9-1-1. It was then that I understood the underpinning of my strong inclination toward inertia. My heart had power over me, not the other way around. If I wanted to survive with this valve-repaired, aged, transplanted heart, I would have to heed even its most subtle warnings.

So now I sit. Just sit.

All day. All night.

I don't reach for the *New York Times* that Scott brings along each morning.

I don't open my laptop.

Even television has quickly become too much.

But I can still engage in conversation, thank goodness, because this is what fills my days with all of these friends. And at night, if I have trouble settling down after a run of pacemaker firings, I lie here and just listen.

Right now, I'm listening to Joy—to the great sound she makes when she sleeps. It is exactly the sound you might expect from her—kind of a smiley, contented *mmm*. I heard it for the first time by chance some seven or eight years ago while staying overnight at her apartment in Bethesda. Passing by her bedroom door early in the morning, a distinct sound in triplicate stopped me on the spot—*mmm, mmm, mmm*. I peeked inside and glimpsed my slumbering friend tucked under a perfectly puffed duvet. A pair of plush slippers lay centered on a white linen mat beside the bed, and on the night table sat a mug and matching tea cozy decorated in wildflower motif—each of these accessories set in place with intention and style, all special touches that Joy had made *just so*. It seemed to me in that moment that her happy sighs of repose fit naturally with the comfy, lovely surroundings she'd created for herself.

In fact, as I had learned during a tour of her apartment the night before, Joy had selected much of the décor for specific effect: namely, to boost and reinforce her own spirit. Stepping into the foyer, she pointed above our heads to a chandelier made of delicate shells that was, she sighed, "like a sea-spray memory from the Hamptons," where carefree summer days were spent with family. A few stops later, we entered the living room, where a large subway sign hung prominently as wall art. "Notice the train line—the Seven . . ." she bubbled. "Takes me straight from Manhattan to my amazin' Mets!" She had been a superfan since she was a kid.

Moving from room to room, Joy revealed to me with pride and emotion several other décor items that filled her apartment and touched her soul with the warmest, most meaningful symbolism—connecting her to friends, family, and her beloved hometown, New York.

"Your apartment feels like love," I told her early the next morning, trying to strike up light conversation as we climbed into her car for what was sure to be a tense drive into Georgetown. "It's no wonder you make those happy little sounds when you sleep."

Joy stopped at a red light and kept her eyes straight ahead. "Oh, so you heard those. Yeah, I know I make 'em. But they're not happy sounds. They're stress."

"We can't be talking about the same thing. These were snuggly, cozy *mmm*s, like if you were drinking warm cocoa."

"Nope. Comes out at night when I let my guard down. Sometimes the sound wakes me up. It's angst."

"Nah, can't be. What *I* heard is—"

Joy breathed out a loud sigh and I stopped myself midsentence. Her lower lip was quivering.

Joy's appearance can play tricks, even on me.

It's her buoyancy that does it: she's indefatigably up. I've never seen anyone hunt down opportunities for enthusiasm the way Joy does. She'll shout "Brilliant!" at my suggestion that we order two appetizers and split one entrée, and whoosh, I'm riding the wave right along with her.

But it's not fair to say I'd been deceived by Joy's demeanor since my arrival in DC the day prior; I know very well that her steady sparkle has years of effort and honing behind it. This is perhaps the way in which we are most alike, Joy and I—in how hard we've worked for the armor we don each day. We've talked often about the frustrations of putting on such a strong appearance all the time. And yet it has been with each other's ongoing support that we've been able to brick ourselves up mightier and mightier as the years have passed—my wall being a barrier against scary health premonitions, and Joy's a deflector of worries that scratch at her mind as a woman who is single.

We know the signs of each other's brick-wall fissures. Joy's nighttime sound was one—and I'd missed it.

"Fear, right?" I said as we sat at a standstill in traffic on M Street. I knew I could be direct with Joy; she's always up for meeting my frankness with her own. "You're fearful about today."

"I am. And then I start to think about how, if I were married, it might be easier."

"Well, you know what *I* say to that . . ."

She does. It would be a reiteration of our go-to talk, a specific bit of clarity that living with serious illness has shown me. My insights rarely apply to healthy people, but I sensed years ago that this particular one would mean something to Joy.

"We are, all of us, alone," she said, reciting the key tenet we'd hashed out so many times.

"Yes, and even if you had a husband, it would still be *you* on center stage today. Even the most wonderful man couldn't stand in your place."

Joy agreed. As hard as this reality was, she'd long been taking my words to heart—mostly because of Scott, who'd made for an undeniable example. Joy knew firsthand his goodness and kindness; she was among the first friends at law school whom Scott told that he loved me, and the only one he wept with when it became clear that I was dying of heart failure at twenty-five. Joy knows that I have the most extraordinary love, the most devoted, adoring, and caring husband imaginable, and yet she also knows that I've come to the realization that ultimately I am still alone in my illness. Because when your face is covered with a sterile sheet and you're clenching the grooves right out of your molars while a doctor plucks seventeen razor slices from your heart for biopsy, you realize, *I've got only myself to rely on right now . . . It all comes down to me.*

This doesn't take away from the greatness of love, not at all. Rather, it holds love apart and exalts it for what it is: magnificent togetherness that balances out the aloneness that must always be.

"All right, scratch what I said about having a husband with me today." Joy chuckled, sitting up taller at the wheel. "I'm okay, I really am. Even so, I'm beyond thankful that you came all the way to DC for this." She pulled into a parking lot, took a ticket from the machine, and handed it to me. "You hold onto this, okay?"

"Of course."

I followed her to the entrance of a modern office building. An attendant gave the rotating door a push, and we came through together in one compartment. As we walked the length of the lobby a sudden gust of air came up, splaying our silk blouses against our bodies and our bangs from our foreheads. The click-click of our shoes echoed with power and purpose against the marble floor. We looked good. Polished. I'd planned to wear something more casual this morning, until I thought of Scott and the rule he'd made for himself when accompanying me to my brick-wall challenges: *Always dress well because it makes everyone take you more seriously.*

"I think registration is in here," Joy said, opening the door to an office on the ground floor.

I linked my arm through hers as we approached the desk.

"Hello. I'm Joy Ceterra. I'm here for my breast biopsy."

LEJA STANDS ON a chair, reaching as high as she can toward the ceiling while Joy directs her, "Two inches to the left . . . now up, and up some more . . ."

"But I must be on one leg!" she shouts with a giggly lilt, twisting her torso as she rises on tiptoe. "Okay, I try . . ."

"We better not get one of those California earthquakes right now!" I joke. We'd felt a small one at the bungalow a few weeks earlier.

"Ahhh! Don't make me to laugh or I fall!" Her right leg is lifted behind her.

"Right there . . . perfect!" Joy calls out. Leja presses her thumb to the wall, teetering precariously. Joy dashes over with arms outstretched to steady her. "There you go, you got it—and thank you, Leja! You can come down now, that's the last of the high ones. And don't they look fabulous!" The three of us glance around at a job well done: twenty rubber-chicken pushpins set into all four walls at perfectly spaced intervals. Joy surveys the remaining shopping bags scattered on the floor and reaches excitedly into a large white one. "Next, the peace signs!"

We've already put in a full day of redecorating my hospital room. Joy set it all in motion yesterday when she arrived with a small suitcase and several bags from a party store back in DC. She pulled out endless streamers and sparkly feather boas like a magician.

"You're not putting those on the wall?" I said.

"You're right, I'm not . . . *Leja*'s doing it with me!" Joy bubbled, and they set to work at once. By midafternoon, squares of colored construction paper covered much of the ecru paint, and a wide strip of blackboard adhesive ran the length of the dry-erase board beneath the dreaded daily-weight sign. *Let there be . . . a heart!* Joy scribbled in white chalk.

It was a wall-to-wall transformation—Joy-style. Applying the same sensibility to my hospital room as she did to her apartment, Joy aimed not just for visual effect, but also for a shift in aura. My room lacked humor, so naturally she thought, *Rubber chickens!* A kick of kitsch might work some magic too: bring on the luau paraphernalia! The objective was to make the room feel full of enormous love, like cross-country friendship and better times to come and the biggest hug that had ever been laid on me.

"But we're not there yet," Joy said, peeved and frowning, when yesterday's California sun started to set. Flopping down on her cot to rest after hanging and adjusting and coordinating just about everything in those shopping bags, she looked around—*hmmm, hmmm*—until inspiration struck. Within minutes there was action (decided upon by a quick caucus out of my earshot); Leja grabbed her sweatshirt and was off to the store—"for the secret we do for you!" she said, giddy to be so very in on it.

I still don't know what that secret is. One night and most of one day have since passed, and the decorating continues without any sign of a big reveal. Leja and Joy reach into a bag to retrieve the peace signs now, and my cell phone rings. "Probably Scott," I say, figuring he's on his way with a pizza for all of us. "Oops, no . . . it's my Columbia doctor."

Joy nods. "Go ahead . . ."

Leja grabs her purse, adding, "I go to bungalow. Skype with my daughter now . . ."

"Hello?" I lie back in bed. Joy unfurls a lavender fleece blanket and tucks me in like a mummy from shoulders to toes. "Thanks for calling, Dr. Davis . . ."

He's responding to an email I sent to him a few days ago about the total artificial heart. Even though he made it clear to me back in New York that my cardiac care must be kept strictly under Dr. Kobashigawa's direction while I'm a patient here (and the Cedars team has since reiterated that), instinct nudged me to reach across the country for his viewpoint on this. Dr. Davis has been my transplant cardiologist for almost twenty-six years: it seems unnatural to rely solely on a new doctor's opinion when making such a weighty decision as whether to agree to a motor-driven temporary heart. In the moments of greatest uncertainty and dread, there is something to be said for history and habit and the comfort that comes from an utterly familiar voice on the other end of a phone.

In his usual curt way, Dr. Davis skips all pleasantries. "You have a question," he says.

"Yes, thanks for calling. Dr. Kobashigawa says I'm getting much worse and he recommends that I sign a paper saying I will do an artificial—"

"A total artificial heart. I am familiar with Cedars's use of them, yes."

Joy gets up on the chair now, hanging psychedelic peace-sign placards with tape.

"Yeah. So, here's how I feel about it. I'm in a tough spot because if I say no—"

"Don't."

"What?"

"Don't do it."

"Don't do the artificial heart—or don't say no to it?"

"Don't do the artificial heart."

"Oh, hmmm, all right. I was leaning that way anyway. But is there a particular reason . . . ?"

"Don't. Okay?"

He means to end the discussion right here, I know. But I push on. "Can you please tell me why?"

"I wouldn't."

"You wouldn't tell me why—or you just wouldn't do it . . ."

"Don't do it. An artificial heart is not for you, Amy. Okay? Bye." He hangs up in typical abrupt Dr. Davis fashion.

And yet, unlike most calls I've had with him over the years, this one leaves me feeling immediately and oddly satisfied. For better or worse, Dr. Davis has stood at the helm of every one of my medical moments and, I imagine, felt the ground shake beneath him. Any advice he gives me—I recognize now more than ever—is uniquely grounded not only in the person and patient he knows me to be, but also in the medical trials I've faced and how close to the end of my rope they've landed me. Stone-cold as Dr. Davis may be, the man gets me.

Dr. Kobashigawa simply can't know me that way. Not yet, anyway. For all his incomparable geniality at my bedside each morning, he doesn't see the shadowy history behind my eyes, no matter how deeply or earnestly he looks into them. My tears, to him, seem only of the moment, and my choices contemporaneous. It is one thing for a doctor to simply read *breast cancer/double mastectomy* in my chart and quite another for him to get an emergency call from my breast doctor on a Friday afternoon, hearing, "I want to talk with you before I speak with Amy. It's cancer . . ." and then immediately lining up a surgeon and an operating room, coordinating all the next steps in swiftest succession, as Dr. Davis did. He wasn't at all sure that I would agree to any kind of breast cancer treatment, but he was absolutely certain that if I did, I would want to move forward with uncommon speed.

This is what compelled me to email Dr. Davis about the artificial heart: the deep, dependable roots of his insight into the big picture, the medical me. And in the definitiveness of what he just told me over the phone, Dr. Davis has shown again that he is as anchored as I am by these roots.

An artificial heart is not for you, Amy.

It sure isn't. And he is the only doctor who can know this right away and for certain.

Lowering the cell phone from my ear, I sense that I'm scowling and smiling at the same time. Joy sees the change in my face and puts down the roll of Hawaiian skirt grass that is fast becoming my new window trim. "You okay, Ames?"

I nod absently. "Weird, though. My New York cardiologist . . . he just barked an order and hung up on me, and it was sort of, uh . . . *great.*"

"Barked? Doesn't sound too great."

"Strange, right? But just this once, I was totally up for the guy telling me exactly what to do. I think I'm getting weary, Joy. Too much to figure out and think about . . ."

"You're exhausted. Hell, I'm exhausted just from last night. Your heart was pacing every forty-five minutes." She collapses into a chair beside me.

"It's gotten a lot worse, I guess."

Joy leans all the way forward and lands her elbows on my bed, her head dropping between them. "What's going to happen when it starts coming every fifteen minutes? You won't sleep at all! And I'll tell you this—you can't be strong if you can't get your sleep. We need to find a way. Lauren spoke with Justin about it . . ." Justin is my favorite nurse.

"Ha, of course she did! About sleep drugs, right? Justin says there's an order in my chart for Valium if I want it. Dr. Lunchbox wrote it."

"How about trying some tonight? It'll be nice. We can get Justin in here and he can talk you to sleep."

"And *you'll* have some eye candy." I grin, swatting her forearm.

"He certainly wins the hunky-night-nurse award, you ain't kiddin'."

"Maybe he's single. Did you see a ring?"

"We were talking about Valium, Ames."

"And I changed the subject."

"I take that as a no, then?"

"Right."

Joy brings up her pointer finger. "You want to be in control," she instructs. "I get it. Hell, my dad calls me Iron Lady—Margaret Thatcher—and I can't say I mind. I'm all for being strong. But taking Valium is not weak. It's actually *control*—over the sleep issue. Be strong and take control of that."

"I'm not a Valium person and you know it."

The drug's mechanism (tranquilizing me so that I might perceive the pacemaker's fiery pain to a lesser degree) goes against everything I've learned about the dangers of compromising one's awareness in a medical setting. As an inpatient over the years, I've had nurses hand me dosing cups with other patients' medicine in them—*whoops!* I've been on biopsy tables where a doctor stabs at my neck, struggling to thread the catheter into a vein, until, finally, I give him some direction, saying, "I'm superficial" (a polite, medically correct way of saying, *Try closer to the surface before stabbing me again, please*). My longstanding aversion to sedation isn't just about gaining a tougher skin with each medical challenge that I face head-on; it is also how I spot errors and save myself from harm.

Joy puts her hand against my cheek. "Amy. I think you've got to let go a little bit here. You can't function without sleep. You'll lose your mind."

My throat tightens as I realize a frazzled brain can be as risky as a sedated one. *What if I've lost my mind already?*

I steer my thoughts into immediate poem retrieval (a challenging one—E. E. Cummings) and launch into silent, rapid-fire recitation for reassurance:

Somewhere I have never travelled, gladly beyond any experience, your eyes have their silence: in your most frail gesture are things which . . . uh . . . things which

Scott walks in just then and distracts me from my memory lapse. I expect him to be toting a pizza box, but instead he's carrying a stack of papers.

Joy whispers to me, winking, "We'll talk about this later . . . with Justin."

"Amy, honey, I've got something you're going to love," Scott announces. "And before I show you, I have to give all credit to Joy. This is all her idea and doing."

"And Leja's!" Joy says, "She did the printing part . . ."

"Is this the big surprise?" I ask.

"Yup, yup! Let's see what ya got, Scotty." She takes the papers from him and begins thumbing through. "Wonderful, wonderful! Ha! Oh, and this one is priceless!"

"What!" I call out. Joy turns the page around so I can see: it's a close-up of my niece in a full-body banana costume with only a small cutout for her face. "Abby!" I shout, laughing.

"Yeah, she got the spirit right. So, I sent a mass email this morning asking everyone to take a loony selfie and send it to me ASAP"—Joy continues to look through the pile—"but I see here that some of these, well . . . not enough loon. Still great, though. And so many! Hey, here's another funny one . . ."

A friend with eyes bugged out, nostrils flared, and with her hair covered in paste and folded into aluminum foil sections.

"At the hair colorist!" Joy cackles. "Brilliant! There are a few more gems in here. But that's all I'm going to show you right now, my friend, because this whole pile is going up *right there*." She points to the wall directly across from my hospital bed. "Let's get started! If you'll give me a hand, please, Scott . . ."

"At your service!"

I lie back and watch them work. Down come half a dozen pink feather boas and a few peace-sign placards. "To be relocated!" Joy calls out. Medical tape in hand, Scott marks and re-marks boundaries according to Joy's eyeball estimations; it takes them a while, and I feel my initial excitement turn to lethargy.

"I think I'll close my eyes for a few minutes."

"Oh, good, honey," Scott says, coming up alongside my bed. He strokes my hair as I curl up beneath the throw blanket. I sense that I'm mumbling—*It's hard to breathe . . . so, so hard*—but all he hears are drowsy sighs that he mistakes for my drifting off. "You sleep now, my love, you sleep," he says.

But I won't. If I let myself really relax, my pulse will drop like it does at night, and my pacemaker will fire through my chest. When I said, *I'll close my eyes*, I meant only that. My mind and body need to remain awake and active to keep the pain from coming.

As I lie still and preserve my energy, Scott and Joy confer quietly.

"She's *so* tired," Joy says.

"I know."

"It's worrisome. I'm going to try to get her to take a Valium tonight. Maybe Justin can help. I put in a request for him to be Amy's nurse again tonight. Lauren told me I could do that."

"That's great. But Amy is, you know, headstrong. Chances are she's not going to take it. Maybe I should sleep here tonight and you can stay with Leja at the bungalow and get some rest."

"No way, buster! My place is on that cot. Period. Now—which photos do we want on the top line?"

"You're a good friend, Joy. Amy is lucky."

"And I'm lucky too. I want to be here. If I can make one small bit of difference to you and Amy when you're slogging through this wait, it's worth a few nights without sleep."

"Well, maybe Amy will give you a break tonight and try a Valium."

Give Joy a break.

I should, shouldn't I?

So many people are doing all they can for me—friends, family, doctors, nurses, night and day, every day—and what do I do for them? Measure my pee? Try to eat a little something? All I do is take, take, take. My responsibilities, other than keeping up the fight for life, are nonexistent. I'm too sick for anyone to expect anything from me. But that doesn't mean I shouldn't be giving them anything.

A break.

Yes. I can try, at least, by putting aside my aversion to sedatives.

Joy would be happy. Scott too. Justin would feel gratified, as would the prescriber of the drug, young Dr. Lunchbox. By simply swallowing one pill, I can perform a very apparent act that's giving and loving and kind.

I won't gain any additional sleep by it, though.

Medical logic tells me so: If Valium is meant to bring my neurological and physiological activity down to a sleepy whisper, then it will also slow down my pulse rate. This means that the benzodiazepine wallop will actually wind up increasing the number of fiery pacing episodes overnight. Surely the doctors and nurses recognize this. Are they figuring the Valium will reduce the pain I feel during pacing episodes enough so that, even if they come at greater frequency, I can better manage them? I don't buy it.

I'm left, then, with a choice: use my own medical reasoning to spare myself additional suffering, or simply do what is being asked of me by my medical team and the people I love. I mull this over, keeping my eyes closed.

"All right . . . on the top we've got your parents, and then Ann, Gary, dog Winnie, dog Milo, Deirdre and her two boys, and, uh . . . who's that?" Scott asks.

"My niece. Amy helped her prepare for her seventh grade chorus solo last month . . ."

"Middle line—Griffen, Lily, Val, Casey with two friends and—oh, nice—a pitcher of beer . . ."

I feel that tug again: *All this love coming at me, but what am I giving in return?*

Death be not selfish, right?

Scott's cell phone rings; it's the pizza delivery. He tells Joy he's going down to the lobby to pick it up. His sneakers squeak from the room.

I open my eyes to slits, just enough to peek without Joy noticing. Through eyelash haze, I see Joy up on a chair smoothing a long piece of tape across an expanse of photo collage. She lowers herself to the floor, takes a few steps back to regard the whole, and then climbs up again to make small adjustments. *Down, up, down, up*—she repeats the process a few more times, aiming for perfect symmetry and positioning. Joy has faith in the placement of objects. Surroundings, as Joy sees them, are not merely suggestive; if chosen with heart and mind, they actually speak directly to you. A span of corkboard, when accented with rubber-chicken pushpins, prompts laughter. A drab window trimmed up in grass-skirt fluorescence beckons you toward the sun. And a wall covered in beloved smiles plus a couple of furry tails and a human-size banana—well, if it's curated by my friend Joy, then it becomes a wall of love.

I pop my eyes open to fully appreciate the scene. "Wow!"

Joy plummets into a squat on the chair, hand flat against her chest. I've startled her. "Whoa," she says. "Now that you've given me a heart attack . . . *Oof*, I shouldn't say that!"

We laugh.

"Really, Joy—wow. This wall is . . . well, *all* the walls, really . . . you've done something amazing here."

"Nah, nah, stop. I'm just the paper hanger." She sits beside me on the bed and exhales long and tired. "It's the faces that make that wall, and they all came from the people you see up there. I sent a group email and, like, ten minutes later, I got the most enthusiastic response. The selfies, the kindest notes . . . they poured in. Everyone wants to do something for you, Amy. *Everyone.*"

Scott walks in carrying a cardboard box. "Oh, sweetie, you're up. Good! I've got a pizza here, but I'm happy to run out and get you a yogurt if you prefer, or a bagel, or—"

"Pizza's great," I say, even though my fluid-filled belly probably won't be able to stand a slice. My response to Scott is pure reflex; Joy's words still echo in my head—*everyone wants to do something for you*—and I'm feeling the weight of how I take, take, take.

There's little recompense in a few bites of pizza. But there's more of it, I know, in two and a half milligrams of Valium.

Maybe I'll try it tonight after all.

I SWALLOW THE little yellow pill.

Joy turns off the lights and moves swiftly into distraction mode. "Now tell me, Justin, where do you live exactly?"

This is Justin's third night with us. Joy has already made him her pal and has insisted that he confirm that we're his favorite from among the three rooms assigned to him, saying, "Come on, Justin, who's better than Amy and me?" We are, after all, decades younger than the yellow-socks folks we've spied on our hallway strolls. And now, with the redecorated sleepover party pad, as we've started to call it, Justin has all the more reason to stop in during the night shift, take a seat, and chat with us girls.

He lowers himself into the Lauren chair by the door. "Silver Lake," he answers. "It's about twenty-five minutes east of here. We've got a little garden apartment."

"Oh, so it's *we*, is it? You married, Jus?" Joy says.

Jus? I forget the pill for a minute and settle in to watch the terrific spectacle of Joy reeling a new friend all the way in; she does it with such precision and ease. It's something to see—and learn from.

"I live with my girlfriend, Jeanie, and actually I'm going to propose to her next week."

"Amy, did you hear! Don't fall asleep just yet! I'm about to delve into the life of our fave night nurse. So, Justin . . . you have a ring?"

He flashes a California-white smile. For the first time, I see dimples . . . and those arms, shown off nicely by the short-sleeve Cedars top he's got on. Why didn't I notice this yesterday? I'm on the verge of hooting, *Nice biceps!* but laughter comes out instead. "Sorry," I say, "feelin' a little, ah . . . *light*." Joy pops her eyes at me.

Justin is unfazed. "Bought the ring just two days ago, as a matter of fact. Want to see a picture?" He reaches into his pocket for his cell phone.

"Of course we do!" Joy says, rising from her cot and padding around to the other side of my bed. Justin turns the screen toward her, and she peers at the small image. "Ooh. Is that a marquise cut? Lemme see up close . . ." She squats down beside him, and the cell phone illuminates her eyelashes and the curve beneath her bottom lip. Through a gauzy haze, colors appear matte and oversaturated to me now—I think I see a halo and it's yellow. Or is that gold? Joy is a fresco painting.

"Take a look at my friend here, isn't she something?" I say, sensing little division between my thoughts and words. "And she has the softest skin, I swear. Joy, roll up your sleeve so Justin can feel you."

What am I saying?

It's got to be the Valium . . . or I think so, anyway. It's hard to tell if it has kicked in all the way. I've only taken this drug a few times before, very early on after my first transplant at Columbia. Back then, protocol for annual-exam angiograms included 2.5 milligrams of Valium along with one 25-milligram tablet of Benadryl—a double whammy intended to ease anxiety during the procedure and induce much-needed sleep

afterward. The mechanism to ensure sufficient closure after comple-
tion of the procedure was time spent lying completely flat (a minimum
of eight hours) with a sandbag weight placed atop the femoral artery
access. Better to be sleeping through the irksome, motionless hours
on one's back—and better, also, to be giggling silly at the doctor's lame
jokes while he cuts into your groin.

I took those pills without protest and enjoyed them. I was in my
twenties—a novice patient who didn't know I could refuse when a
nurse handed me one pink pill and one yellow. I also hadn't yet learned
that remaining completely alert and participatory was the safest way to
be in a medical setting, no matter the recommended sedative protocol.
But then new methods for groin closure came along, and patients were
able to get up and out of the hospital after just an hour or so of lying
flat. Long-acting Valium and Benadryl were replaced by short-acting IV
drugs like Versed (the forgetting drug), and that's when I found my
voice as a self-advocating patient and said, "No sedation."

And now, tonight, I've asked for Valium.

In the absence of the added Benadryl kick, I don't know what the
ratio of giggle to slumber might be. But for sure, I am not going to be
at my vigilant, focused best.

"I feel stupid," I say. "And I don't like it."

Joy shifts her attention away from Justin. "You're all right. Just roll
with it."

I start singing under my breath, *"You just roll with it, baby . . . Come
on and just roll with it, baby* . . . Remember that song? Eighties. Steve
Winwood. Fire Island weekend. I was at this bar with Jill, or more like
I was at the bar with Jill's boobs, because they were like two giant guy-
magnets and I was invisible! *Ha-ha-ha-ha* . . . But wait, wait, that's
not funny. It's serious. But also funny, right? I was at a bar with Jill's
boobs!"

"Uh-oh," Joy says, raising her eyebrows at Justin. "Ah, Justin—you
sure you gave her a sleep aid and not a loony bird pill?"

"Affects people differently," he whispers beneath my giggling.

"Sometimes they get real loose at first . . . then sleepy." Trying to meet my eyes, he raises his voice. "Amy, you feeling all right?"

"Yeah," I say, sensing my eyes unfocused and soft. "But I'm not happy . . . I'm not all here." My words are a little slurred and it scares me. I shoot an anxious glance at Joy. "I can't watch out for myself if I'm like this . . ."

"Stop that thought right there," Joy insists. She hands Justin his phone and comes to sit beside me on the bed. "There's nothing for you to do now except sleep."

"But the problem with sleep is this," I say, working hard to clear my head of the thick syrupy languor. "Once I'm asleep, the pacemaker is going to kick in, just like always—don't you think so, Justin? Why didn't Dr. Lunchbox think of that? It makes sense, right? It makes sense." I'm prattling and I know it, but words and thoughts are sticking together now and I have no will to separate them.

"We'll soon find out. Let's hope the Valium will help you sleep through the pacing," he replies.

"*Nooooo*. Not going to happen. Justin. Listen! If a sledgehammer hits you over the head while . . . oh, wait . . . funny! I said *sledgehammer*. Isn't that a Steve Winwood song too? What is this, eighties radio trivia night? Oh, never mind. I'm an idiot on this drug! You know I'm afraid of being all *la-di-da* out-of-my-right-mind, Joy. And what if the Valium slows my breathing? My lungs are full of failure, uh, I mean, fluid . . . uh, I can die if things slow down too much . . ."

She grips my hands tight and shakes them like horse reins. "I know what you're thinking. I know what you fear. And that's why I'm right here beside you. I'm going to sit in that chair with my eyes on you all night, just like I said I would."

I nod with relief and start to let my heavy eyes close.

Justin's eyebrows shoot up. "All night? No, no, no, you need to sleep, Joy. *I'm* the one who stays up all night. That's my role." His whisper is softer now, perhaps in hopes that my closed eyes mean I'm drifting into sleep.

Joy lowers her voice as well. "I promised Amy that if she takes the Valium, I'll stay awake and keep watch over her. I figure I'll take some notes, write down how many times the pacemaker fires and how long it takes to get her pulse above eighty. I'll watch her breathing . . ."

"The monitor does that. It'll let us know if she's not getting air. You don't have to do that."

"I do, Justin. You don't understand how afraid Amy is and what a big deal this is for her to take a sedative. The girl would do her heart transplant surgery awake if she could."

He gets up from his chair. "All right. If it's quiet on the floor to-night, I'll try to stop in and take over for fifteen minutes so you can sleep a little. And keep in mind you *can* rely on the monitor, like we do for all our patients on this floor."

Joy tells him she understands, but wouldn't feel right letting a ma-chine take care of me, not after making a promise to stay awake. "And don't worry about me getting sleep. I'm fine. Plenty of time to snooze on the plane home tomorrow."

My lips move and a few syllables come out. "That's my Iron Lady," is what I mean to say, and I hope that Joy hears.

She sits on the chair beside me. I inch my body to the edge of the bed and extend my arm out to feel her there. Joy takes my hand and, finally, I give in.

The wall she built today has inspired mine to come down.

All right, Valium. I'm yours.

IT'S SEVEN A.M. and Joy reads her notes out loud. "Let's see now," she says, lifting a sheet of lined paper in front of her face. Yellow high-lighter marks show through the page, telling me that she has already reviewed her data carefully and that what I am about to hear is the pre-sentation of a reasoned argument.

"First, the *not*-great news—you were up with pacemaker pain six times."

"Told you. Sledgehammer to the head will wake you every time."

"Not *every* time, and this leads me to the better news. You actually slept through pacing at two thirty and again at three fifteen." She told me she saw it on the monitor, which I had taught her to decipher over the last three nights. "I watched your pulse drop . . . it slid down to something like fifty. The EKG got all squiggly—that was the pacing—but you stayed asleep. As a whole, I'd rate the night as Valium success-*ish*."

"And I'd call it a period from hell." Somewhere after midnight I woke with cramps, and sure enough, I was bleeding. Surprisingly, the severe state of my heart failure did not keep my period from coming on time. What it did instead was bring it forth with a vengeance. I hadn't experienced such a heavy flow or contraction-like cramps since high school. "The pain is worse this morning."

"You sure don't show it. Want some Advil?"

"Not allowed. It interacts with transplant medicines."

"Can't you take just . . ."

We hear someone push open the door with a "Morning, morning." It's Dr. Kobashigawa. "Hello, hello." He shakes my hand, then Joy's. "I think I'll take a seat before examining you, if that's all right." He asks me how my night was, and I tell him I woke with a terrible period.

"It's bringing so much extra pain," I say, hugging my thighs to my chest for a few seconds before breathlessness forces me to let them go.

"Can she take, maybe, just one Advil?" Joy asks.

Dr. Kobashigawa flashes his warm smile. "Oh nooo. That would be very dangerous for her kidneys."

I figure I'll try to get by with some Tylenol. But the pain is coming in waves now, sharper and deeper with each one. I can feel my pajama bottoms sopping with blood, and the thought is nauseating. I start to hope this will be one of Dr. K's shorter morning visits.

"I have some good news about your status on the waiting list," he says. "We've been granted an exception for your case, and this makes you a 1A-E as of yesterday. Let me explain . . ."

I try to focus on his words, but the seizing pain distracts me, and I'm not sure how long I can sit and listen.

He tells us that it was necessary to submit paperwork justifying my 1A-E status (1A is the highest urgency, and E is for an Exception) because the particular manifestations of heart failure from which I suffer, as well as the type of life-sustaining care I'm receiving at Cedars, do not fall squarely within the requirements for this top waiting list tier. Even though my vasculopathy is clearly end-stage and irreparable, the diagnostic snapshot of my heart function (a conglomerate of specific test results, including pressure measurements in the right heart and assessment of the pumping capacity of the left ventricle) does not reflect the severity of my extensive artery disease. "And of course you don't have a Swan in your neck, which is a requirement for 1A," Dr. Kobashigawa adds, "another reason why we needed to get you an exception."

He means Swan-Ganz, a catheter named after the two doctors who invented it (one of them at Cedars) back in 1970. Externally, the device looks like a plastic tube attached to the side of the neck and curled at the top like a memorial ribbon. Beneath the surface, it runs through the jugular vein and into the heart, where cardiac-sustaining medications can be delivered directly and their effects monitored.

"Most of the patients on this floor have a Swan in place," he explains to Joy. "But Amy's condition cannot tolerate the dobutamine that would be administered through it."

"Revs up the heart like a race car. Keeps it beating," I explain. "Although a few cc's of dobutamine would actually kill me."

Dr. Kobashigawa closes his eyes and grins. "You don't mince words. And once again, you are correct."

Another sharp pain grips my pelvis. I feel a gush of blood between my legs.

Oh, crap, I'm going to vomit . . .

"And so, the 1A-E. You're at the top of the list now."

Joy brings her hands together in a single clap. "Fan-tastic! Brilliant!"

He holds up a hand to caution us. "The 1As who've accumulated longer waiting time will have priority," he says. "And then of course we need an antibody match—that's tricky, but I'm going to stay optimistic." He gets up from his chair and steps forward to examine me.

Hold it together, Amy. Don't puke on the guy. Think saltine crackers . . . saltine crackers . . . ginger ale . . .

The stethoscope lands first on my back. "Breathe . . . and again . . ." he instructs. He turns my chin to the left and assesses the throbbing purple vein in my neck. "Never fails to amaze," he says.

"Yeah." I've broken into a sweat. Just a few more seconds while he listens to my heart . . .

Stethoscope to chest now. Pause, pause, pause.

"All right. I will see you, then, tomor—"

"I'm sorry, but I have to throw up!" I lurch forward and he jumps out of the way with a "Whoop!" and heads for the door, promising to get the nurse.

I rush to the bathroom, drop to my knees, and begin heaving.

Within seconds, Joy is kneeling alongside me. She puts her hand on my back while I vomit again and again. When I finish, she grips my arm and helps me to standing, fills a cup with water and steadies me while I rinse. Again, I feel a surge of blood; this time it runs down the inside of my legs, all the way to the floor. "Oh God, I gotta sit down . . ." Joy helps me turn around and sit down on the toilet. She notices that my pajama bottoms are soaked with purplish-red blood; I look down at the mess and start to weep as another wave of pain cuts through my lower abdomen. "I need to . . . get these pants off, but I . . . I'm going to throw up again . . ."

Suddenly there's a basin in front of me; Joy spotted it on a high shelf and landed it on my lap in seconds. She is everywhere at once—an octopus woman with eight arms in motion. "But my pants . . . the blood," I moan, just before another heave.

Her hand returns to my back. "We'll get you cleaned up in a minute. Don't worry." She rubs and rubs in gentle circles. "Shhh . . ."

Soon, the cramping and nausea begin to calm. "I think that's it," I say. She lifts the basin promptly from my lap.

"I'm going to put this just outside the bathroom until I figure out what to do with it," she says, and I watch her bend to place it just beyond the door frame. She pops up and whirls to face me. "Now, those pajama pants . . ."

Joy kneels in front of me. I try to place my thumbs under my pajama-bottom waistband, but I'm weak and shaking. She takes over at once, sliding the saturated flannel past my knees and feet. I look down and see that my blood-soaked underwear still clings midthigh, but I've got my hands on either side of the toilet seat now and I feel I may collapse if I lift them. "I can't . . ." I whimper.

"I'm on it," she assures me, and sets to removing my underwear in a succession of small, sticky tugs. She tosses it along with the pajama pants into the shower stall, then steps quickly over to the sink. Soon, she's standing in front of me with a wet towel. "It's warm," she says. "Want to clean up down there?"

I glance at my blood-smeared thighs; I desperately want to clean them, but my body is still weak and trembling. This violent menstrual period is a new challenge that has rendered me immediately helpless, but I find myself easing into the hands that care for me. With the seamless presence of loving friends week after week, ceding some of my independence is starting to feel like an act of gratitude.

I don't even reach for the towel. "I . . . I don't know if I can."

Her response is instantaneous: "Let me help." I accept gladly.

It was only two months ago that I scoffed at Joy's offer to sleep in my bedroom back in New York. But now here I am in California, unfathomably exposed, and I've invited this same friend to lay eyes and hands on a most private part of me, tending to the task of cleaning my bottom half with the gentle thoroughness of a mother.

She tosses the used towel onto the shower floor and heads to the closet for some fresh clothes. "I don't need a shirt, this one's clean," I call out.

"You need a shirt. Change up your outfit, change the mood of the day." She steadies me as I stand up to slip on the clothes. "Period from hell, be gone!" she commands.

And why not? Joy's intentions wield power here. For the past four days, I've watched them transform every corner of my hospital room, setting some of the horror back on its heels and proving once again her credo that atmosphere matters, not only for me in the wake of blood and vomit in the bathroom, but for all who enter this setting of galloping heart disease throughout the day and night. Cedars staff have been stopping in more often and staying longer now that Joy and her décor are in place; nurses plop down in Lauren's chair, let out a sigh, and tell us, "*Ahhh*, this room transports me . . . Mind if I just sit here a bit?" And by the time they leave, Joy has made a new friend for herself—and for me. Her attention is fairy dust.

I can feel its magic on me as I lie here now, reclining on the bed with a soft blanket over my legs, cleaned and cleared of the early-morning ordeal that Joy has placed tidily behind us. I reach into my drawer for my Tylenol stash, swallow two Extra Strength caplets, and begin again the day that she's already made better for me.

"You handled that really well," she says.

"I'd say it was *you* who did the handling . . . or the pretty darn disgusting multitasking, really. I'm sorry you had to see all that."

"See what? I was in action mode. Constant movement. No time for being grossed out. I will accept no sorries. Sorry!"

"So then—what? I should just say thank you?"

"I know you would have done the same for me, you big goofball. And hey, you've already done wonderful things for me, if you want to start comparing."

She brings up the breast biopsy from years ago. The pathology result turned out to be benign, but the specter of an alternative outcome shook her to the core. We had a long talk together the night before the procedure, and Joy had shed rare tears of panic and dread. "What happens if I have cancer? How will I manage chemotherapy?" she wondered.

Joy reminds me now what I said in response: "You told me, 'Then, you'll come live with us until you're well.' I felt safe because I knew you meant it." She insists I've provided other refuge as well, and begins to revisit the ways I've run reliable interference against some of the less obvious anxieties of her single life, including times I stayed on the phone with her when the cable or repair man came through the door. "Honey, what time do you think you'll be home for dinner?" she would say as I played husband to her housewife so that the eavesdropping intruder wouldn't know she lived alone. And there was a particular rough patch back when we were in our thirties, Joy reminds me, when she would go on a trip and couldn't help but think, *How long will it take anyone to realize if I don't make it back home again?* Sending me an email with flight numbers, dates, and times gave her a feeling of security.

"None of those things involved wiping up period blood," I point out.

"I call it even," she says. "And don't try to tell me that I did the work in that bathroom—because it was you. You were amazing. So strong and focused—you didn't even throw up on me! We were a great team in there."

Great team. Amazing, strong, and focused.

That's what Lauren said last week.

I wonder how specific the nightly emails have become. Do they now include sample statements for helpful conversation or praise? It can't be a coincidence that Lauren and Joy are using the same words. There's a conspiracy of lauding going on, and curiously, I don't mind.

Over the years, my friends have learned to refrain from complimenting me on how well I abide my body ills. They've seen me take quick offense to pats on the back for actions, deeds, or behaviors that would not be worthy of attention in a healthy individual. But now, here's Joy reminding me of the long history of reciprocity in our friendship and connecting me to my stronger, more giving self, and I'm uplifted by it. And when she tells me that I vomit with good aim and that, boy oh boy, can I withstand a spate of killer menstrual contractions—I'm surprised to find myself thinking, simply, *Thanks for saying so.* Commendable action has a new measure here in this hospital room, and so I respond to it in a new way; because the trials of my body are displayed conspicuously, I do not feel affronted by praise for how I deal with them. Instead, I feel fortunate that all my girlfriends seem intent not only on pointing out the best of my daily endeavors, but also on ensuring that the next visitor on the schedule does the same. They figured out—even before I did—that this is what I need.

Although these women arrive individually and sleep on the cot by themselves, they are linked, I now see, by a strong, supportive chain. They are never without each other in this retransplant effort, and I am never without the whole group of them, regardless of who may sit beside me on any given day.

Are we all—all of us—alone, then?

I look at the photo collage on the wall.

I'm not so sure anymore.

"Now it's time for me to go clean myself up," Joy says, gathering her toiletry case and towel. She will go to the hallway bathroom rather than use mine here in the room, and it is by her own declaration that she (and all visitors) must do so. "You don't need everyone's germs," was how she put it, proposing a Joy Amendment to the bathroom procedure a few days ago. I imagine she's put it into writing in the group email, codifying it into law.

She steps into the hallway, and I reach into my night table drawer for the drawing pad Jody brought for me. I pull out a red colored pencil and write in large letters a quote I'd memorized back in college. Yeats. It was just one of many lines that struck me back then, but now I have an eerie feeling that I was meant to find it, to learn it, and to be alive to use it just this way.

I get out of bed and muster enough strength to push a chair up to the wall of selfies. I climb onto the seat shakily, Scotch tape in one hand and the sheet of drawing paper in the other. By the time Joy walks in, I've barely got enough breath to speak. "Can you . . . tell me if this . . . is the center?" I place my hand on the spot I think may be the middle.

"I think so, ah . . ." She steps back from it. "Down a bit and over to the . . . *Wait!* Get down from there! Let me do that, you silly!"

We switch places and I direct her. Joy presses some tape to the wall and stands motionless, staring for a few long seconds. When she turns around, her eyes are welled with tears.

"That's perfectly beautiful," she says.

I look up at my handwriting, nestled now among the many, many faces:

Think where man's glory most begins and ends,
And say my glory was I had such friends.
                                        —Yeats

From: Joy Ceterra
Subject: The Wall of Love
Date: April 17, 2014 at 11:50 AM
To: Jill Dawson, Lauren Steale, Valerie Yablon, Jane Keller, Robin Adelson, Jody Solomon, Ann Burrell, Leja Babic

Thanks everyone for sending your photos so quickly. Along with the others I've received so far, they've turned the drab hospital wall to color and love for Amy. I wish you could have seen the big smile on her face at the moment of my big reveal! Lights, camera . . . Wall of Love! (See photo below: it's a work in progress . . . more photos coming in day by day, so when you're here, please continue to mount them—Scotch tape in Amy's night table drawer.)

Sad to say, I am leaving today. But Val arrives shortly to keep the friend chain going and the love flowing. We've had good moments and not so good moments here this week, but most importantly, together with wonderful Scotty and the amazing daily presence of Jack and Jody, we've filled Amy's days with comfort, warmth and even some laughter too.

Next project on deck: Let's get our girl a freakin' heart—NOW!

Wishing you . . . JOY

8

made the transplant pharmacist cry. Becky (I think her name is) scurried out of my room a few seconds ago, distraught, and Scott—always the good guy—went after her to apologize.

Sorry that Amy can't just let it go, he's probably telling her in the hallway right now. Soon, I suppose, he'll step back in here with a disappointed frown, saying, *You could have handled that differently*, and I'll have to respond—a challenge I'm likely to flub, because while, yes, I could have taken another tack with Becky just now, the quiet truth is I'm sort of glad I didn't.

Not that I meant to draw tears from her; she has been nothing but well-meaning while standing among the horseshoe formation of transplant-team white coats at the foot of my bed each morning. But to have *just let it go* in this situation would have resurrected the submissive, terrified girl I was at the time of my first transplant. Instead, to have the smarts to know when ground is worth standing in a medical setting—and to be courageous enough to stand upon it and speak cogently, even when wearing a hospital gown open to the back—is the mark of a self-assured patient and woman.

That's how I see it, anyway. To Scott, though, the scene that just took place is simply a manifestation of my going overboard. This means I've got about thirty seconds to decide whether I'm going to defend my stance when he steps back in here to challenge it.

I ASKED A question about vitamin C—that's what started this whole thing. Becky was nice enough to remain behind to answer it after the heart transplant cadre moved on to the next patient room. "Happy to check for you," she said, and started clicking the keyboard on the Cedars staff computer mounted beside my bed. She asked to see my hospital bracelet to scan in my patient ID, and instead of offering her my wrist I recited the number from memory: 601 056 2852.

"Never seen a patient do that before—kind of cool!" She gave her shag haircut a quick toss, jostling beaded earrings that grazed her neck. I thought she was kind of cool. We engaged in some small talk—*interesting décor in here . . . sort of* Hawaii Five-0 *meets Marcia Brady*—until my file came up on the screen. Becky read aloud while scrolling through my medication list, "I see you're still taking the immunosuppressives they had you on at Columbia. Cyclosporine, Imuran, prednisone . . ."

"Old-fashioned, I know. I'm a relic."

She had her eyes straight ahead on the screen, keeping up perfunctory conversation while skimming the dense pages. "We'll be bringing all your meds into the modern age after your transplant. Now . . . um . . . you asked me about whether you can take . . . Oh, wait a minute . . ." She zooms in on some words that elicit a big smile. "Ooh, I see that you're going to be part of our eculizumab study . . . wonderful!"

"Ecu-lizumab?"

"Yeah. Name's a mouthful, right? I don't blame you if you can't pronounce it. I'm talking about the experimental treatment for your antibodies. You're going to be part of our NIH study."

What?

I'd heard a little bit about the study from Dr. Kobashigawa a few days earlier, and someone from the Cedars medical research team dropped off a thick binder filled with detailed information for my review. But this intravenous drug with the mouthful name was a chemotherapy of sorts and had serious side effects, including a significant risk of meningitis. Were I to participate, these treatments were not imminent (they wouldn't kick in until the time of my transplant surgery). But I had already undergone another potent antibody remedy when I first arrived in California (bortezomib) that posed a risk of blood infections and death. The bortezomib treatments involved a series of direct injections into my belly and many of hours of antibody-cleansing plasmapheresis (plasma removal and replacement) through a thick catheter in my neck. Last I heard, though, the post-bortezomib state of my antibodies was not much better than before treatment; my chance of matching with a heart donor still remained at an inauspicious 14 percent. Feeling fortunate, though, for having at least evaded the dangers of bortezomib, I was not eager to risk another go-round with a second type of antibody treatment—especially an experimental one.

"You're sure my name is on the study roster—already?" My voice rises.

She pecks at the keyboard, double-checking. "Yup, here you are!"

I jolt upright in bed. "But how can that be? I haven't said yes!" Pressing my palms against my temples, I begin to reel. "I can't believe this! Am I being steamrolled into the study?"

"No, no. But the team has decided—"

"The team? *I'm* the one who's supposed to choose."

"Of course you are, but—"

"I have a voice!"

"I didn't mean to make you feel—"

"Just because I'm . . . sick . . . it doesn't mean I don't . . . have a say!" I'm choking on emotion now. Scott steps toward the bed and puts his hand firmly on my shoulder—*Easy, let it go* . . .

Not a chance.

Becky just stepped on a land mine twenty-five years in the making. But she can only see the explosion, not its underpinnings. Deep down there are a hundred hard lessons woven into the fuse from my transplant decades. I can't help but be lit by memories—sometimes so many of them combusting at once, I can't tell for sure which one struck the match. But here this morning, I get the sense that one culprit in particular—the earliest in my medical history—may be both the instigator and the scorching eternal flame.

I've come to think of this particular memory as the strawberry shortcut—a lesson that came by way of a pulmonary lab technician who said playfully, "Let's take the strawberry shortcut," when escorting me from the waiting room to the exam suite. It was 1988. I was in my second year of law school, and my doctor wanted to rule out all possible causes of my very apparent breathlessness. Heart problems seemed so much less likely than lung problems in a woman in her midtwenties, so he scheduled a progression of tests that began with pulmonary.

As I followed in the wake of the technician's perfectly pressed white coat, turning and turning again through a seeming maze of narrow hallways, he called back to me over his shoulder a preview of what was to come. Apparently, I would soon be breathing in some—particles? Nuclear particles? I didn't understand—I'd never had even so much as a strep throat culture in my twenty-five years of life—so I obeyed with some trepidation when he placed the clear plastic contraption over my mouth, nose, and a good portion of both cheeks. "We're friends here, aren't we? So just relax into it and breathe deeply," he cooed, and I tried. But there was nothing about inhaling the particles he administered that made me feel friendly or comfortable. He noted my reluctance at once. "Oh, you're going to have to go deeper than that, pretty," he said.

Pretty?

My stomach muscles tightened with angst. I began to shake.

"In . . . and out. In . . . and out," he coaxed, moving his face closer with each round of inhalation and exhalation until his lips and the tip of his nose were in line with mine, pressing up against the plastic.

I closed my eyes and I felt some tears fall. *I'm trapped. My doctor can't make me better unless I do this test. I've got to get through it. Come on, Amy, breathe . . .*

"That's it . . . *niiiice,*" the technician purred. "And again, for me . . ."

When the test was finished, I hurried off the exam table. "Hey there," he said, reaching for the door handle before I could. "How about a kiss for the technician?"

"How about a handshake instead!" I snapped, surprising him with a sudden show of nerve. He murmured something about a hot tamale and grasped my hand.

A few days later, I filed a complaint with the hospital and was told there was nothing they could do since I didn't remember the tech's name. And besides, they told me, "Maybe he was just trying to help you relax."

That was the start of my growing a backbone as a patient. Hell, if the same thing were to happen to me now, I'd respond directly with, *Kiss? How about you kiss your job good-bye!*

Fifty is so much braver than twenty-five, you see.

Though today's situation was quite different, it preyed on some of my greatest medical fears, those that had developed out of the strawberry shortcut incident and countless others over the years: feeling a lack of agency, feeling uninformed, and feeling taken advantage of. And this is why I felt no trepidation this morning when telling the transplant pharmacist that I wanted to speak with her supervisor: Dr. Kobashigawa. She logged out of the screen at once and backed away from the computer. "I'm sorry to see you so upset about this."

"And *I'm* sorry for these stupid tears, but I can't help it. I've learned the hard way never to turn off my brain and hand myself over. I'm not going to agree to ecu—whatever it's called—without reading through the whole binder and making my own decision."

"I understand. But keep in mind we're just trying to help you, Amy. You've got antibodies that are going to pose a danger to *any* donor heart you might receive. You can't be transplanted successfully without eculiz—"

"I *can't?* Are you saying I don't have choice? That I never really had a choice? Who told you *that?* Dr. Kobashigawa?" My fingertips fly to my forehead and I begin tapping, tapping. A rush of panic sweeps through me—*Have I been duped?*

She started toward the door, pulling nervously at the ends of her hair. It was apparent that Becky had let on more than I was meant to hear just yet, and that perhaps she might be in trouble for it. "I'll, um, ask him to come see you."

But the memory match had already struck and ignited. All of a sudden there were words in the air—my words—and they rang calm and clear at first, but then echoed back to me calamitous and full of smoky black, as if tethered to distant fires. Whatever I was saying was not of this moment; it was cumulative—and ablaze: "Wow, Becky, wow, wow, wow. As if I didn't feel out of control to begin with, watching my pulse disappear day after day. *Thanks a lot.* You sure know how to make a dying person feel worse."

"That wasn't my . . . Oh, I *am* sorry!" she squeaked with panic, tears welling in her eyes. She quickly turned away and slipped out the door.

"I MADE THE transplant pharmacist cry."

Val nods a few times in realization. "Ah . . . *now* I get why Scott was all—"

"Yeah."

She didn't understand at first why he greeted her with a brusque good-bye when she arrived from the airport a few minutes ago. "Great. You're here. Now I can go get some work done," he huffed, gathering up a mess of folders and papers. Val stepped to the side as he brushed past with his briefcase unzipped, half hanging off his shoulder. Just short of the doorway, though, he bumped up against his better nature and rebounded from his uncharacteristic rudeness. "Uh, sorry," he said, pivoting to look at Val directly, "I'm in the middle of a work thing. But thank you for coming, thank you! I gotta run—" He was out the door before she could respond.

Val pulls what looks like a bag of chips from her purse now and tosses it on my bed. "So—how bad did you give it to the poor pharmacist?"

I pick up the bag and read the unfamiliar label. "Okra crisps? Seriously?" I open it and crunch into a small, crispy circle. "Not bad—I mean the way I laced into the pharmacist lady wasn't too bad. These chips, however, are *yuck*."

"How about cashews, then? Take some—they're organic! Or dried cherries? I've got apricots too . . ." She pulls out plastic ziplock bags full of snacks. She still stocks her purse like an earth mother of toddlers, even though her two sons are grown.

"You're a walking Whole Foods, aren't you?" I say.

"Trader Joe's. And look what else I got there . . ." She unzips her carry-on bag and pulls out a fluorescent-green spray bottle–fan combo as long as her arm from elbow to fingertips. "I've got the sweats now—isn't that lovely? No, it's awful! I'm dying of heat, whew!" She pumps the bottle like it will save her life. "Oh *God*, when will this *end*!"

"Ah, menopause—I guess."

"I wish it were freaking over already—good grief! You still get your period?"

"Every month. No sweats."

"Get out of here . . ."

"It's my easy, breezy lifestyle and healthy constitution—*ha-ha*." I pluck a few cashews from the bag and pop them into my mouth, shrugging. "So—the pharmacist . . . she made a big mistake and I jumped on it. That's all."

Val wipes her sopping face with the back of her hand. "Jumped—or *pounced*? You say you made her cry, Ames." She lifts a couple of snack bags at once and waves them in front of me. "Here, take some more. I plan on getting lots of nutrition into you this weekend. I talked with Lauren the other night, and she told me you're rail thin. I promised her I'd do something about it."

Since when do you talk with Lauren?

I'm surprised. Val is not part of my friend group in New York. She was my law school roommate and has lived in Durham for some twenty years now. I don't remember introducing Val and Lauren at any point, although I suppose they've become acquainted through the patchwork of information that gets conveyed when I mention one to the other in conversation: *My friend Val's dog has fleas too—I'll ask her what she uses* or *My friend Lauren sent me this article—I think you'd like it.* But now, it seems, the spreadsheet has brought the two of them together in earnest; the nightly emails circulated among the group seem to have progressed the few unacquainted women to friends in the making.

"Well, I hope Lauren told you about my ankles and feet. *They're* not rail thin." I yank up the bottoms of my yoga pants. "Get a load of these babies—a neon sign for end-stage heart failure."

Val gasps. "Ahh!" Pressing her fingertips tentatively against the bloat, she lifts a pained gaze to meet mine. "Oh, Ames!"

"I told you it was bad."

"And I believed you. But to actually *see* it—" She shakes her head, stunned.

Val and I aren't used to seeing the things we describe to each other. The distance between New York and Durham has forced a phone friendship upon us over the last two decades, precluding the in-person interaction that characterized our early years together in the law school dorm, face-to-face for every bowl of breakfast cereal and step out of the shower. And even though we visit every few years and fill in the space between with evening talks (usually with a phone wedged between ear and shoulder while we prepare dinner), the lack of a visual element allows for a skewed imagining of each other that, for better or worse, becomes the reality.

When I hear Val's voice on the phone, I see in my mind's eye a twenty-three-year-old curly-haired girl wearing an oversized NYU Law sweatshirt and a smile made of orange peel (she liked to cram a wide slice of it against her teeth and hold it there until I laughed). And then, without warning, the modern-day Val will send a selfie to my cell phone and—*what?* Long, smooth tresses? "I've been doing keratin hair straightening for two years," she'll explain. All right—but what's with the contemporary sportswear look? "There was a sale on cardigan sweater sets at Neiman's . . ."

Sweater sets? Who is this woman?

But then, the next night, the familiar voice of my old friend will return in customary form—without an accompanying photo—and we're safely back to the land of phone conversations while we sprinkle paprika and garlic salt on our respective chickens, chatting nonstop as we push them into our ovens to roast. "*Please* tell me you bought organic . . ." Val implores before starting up commentary on my vegetable side dishes. ". . . or else you're eating all those hormones and antibiotics!" That's the Val I know so well—by sound and syntax, and by the routine clobbering over the head for my blasé attitude toward poultry selection. *Talk, listen, talk, listen*—all is comfortable between us again.

Now, for the next three days and nights, there will be no telephone to ensure a safe distance between the visual on either end of the call. Here in the hospital, Val and I will have to open our eyes to a friendship that has relied almost exclusively on open ears. I'm a little apprehensive about how we'll do with the change.

"I feel a little woozy," she tells me, withdrawing her hand from the purplish bloat that consumes my anklebone. "Mind if I cover your feet back up?"

"Of course—sorry. Really."

She lowers herself into a chair and launches into another water-bottle-spraying frenzy. "Whoa, sorry, but I might have to put my head between my legs for a few seconds. You know how I get . . ."

I do. After years of Val reporting to me episodes of near or full-out fainting, I figure she suffers from something I've heard doctors call reactive blood pressure, whereby a strong, negative emotion—dread, alarm, disgust, or being just plain grossed out—can easily send her to the floor. A few months ago, she called me to lift her out of embarrassment following a simple blood draw at her internist's office that nearly necessitated smelling salts. "It happened because I didn't eat anything in the morning," she insisted (Val believes strongly that food is the answer to most body ills).

I offer up some of her own medicine now. "How about a few dried cherries? The sugar might help." I put my hand on the back of her bowed head and stroke her hair.

"I'm good, I'm good," she assures me, lifting her head and smiling. "I'll be fine in a minute. Now—let's talk about that pharmacist." She pushes a few cherry bits into her mouth and gestures for me to sit in the chair beside her—a request with attendant risks that she can't anticipate. Val doesn't yet know that when I sit in a chair (feet toward the floor, torso upright), every one of my toes turns gunmetal gray from oxygen starvation.

"Let me just put on some socks first," I say, taking precautions so my friend won't swoon twice. I sit down beside her and begin to recreate the dialogue from earlier this morning.

"So then the pharmacist tells me, 'Sure, I'll check about the vitamin C . . .'"

Val listens for a good long while, closing her eyes and pressing her lips together when I switch to a reedy, high-pitched imitation of Becky's voice.

"'Only trying to help you, Amy . . .'" I chirp.

"She probably *was* trying, although she messed up pretty awful in the delivery," Val says. "But please, continue. Sorry to interrupt." She reverts to all ears, relaxing back against her chair and extending both legs to rest on my bed. Her hands lie palms up in her lap, and she's smiling serenely, as if settling in with a good book.

We have time in this hospital setting. Unusual, uninterrupted time. Full days and nights of no cricking our necks to balance the phone while we chop garlic. No children needing our attention or husbands walking through the door after a long workday—automatic trump cards that, for both of us, result in an immediate *I gotta go* . . . Now it's just us: two friends who haven't had much opportunity to spend an unhurried half hour together in twenty-five years.

But as firmly planted as we are here, and as slow and easy as the moments feel, there is an unspoken awareness of our time together being limited in a different way from ever before. It is not life that will cut our conversation short this time but, rather, the possibility of death. The hourglass is filled with quicksand.

I finish the pharmacist story with flourish: "And then—cue the organ music—Scott shoots me a look—*da-da-DAH!*—and dashes into the hall."

"Okay. So . . ." She sits up straight and looks at me directly. "You were supposed to read through the materials and *then* make a decision about whether to do the antibody treatment. Then the pharmacist essentially says that the choice had been made *for you*—so you react. Nothing wrong with that, although . . . your line about making a dying person feel worse was a little, shall we say, over the top?"

"As I see it now, yeah. I'd take it back if I could—"

"But you can't. And now Scott's mad at you even though, really, you were just sticking up for yourself."

"Exactly."

"And you lost your cool because, when it comes right down to it, you're trying to save your life. Sounds a lot to me like the angiogram you had a few years ago where the doctor screwed up, and you said to him—oh my gosh, what you said to him! Scott was *so* upset with you, remember? But *I* understood . . ."

She did—and better than anyone else, perhaps—because Val possesses impressive insight and empathy into the problems of others. It also helps that she is married to a doctor. When I shared with her a quick overview of the angiogram mishap, she called out to him, "Jeff! What happens if lidocaine gets shot straight into your vein by accident?"

"Who'd *that* happen to?" I heard him answer.

"Amy. During her angiogram at Columbia."

"Dangerous stuff. She could've stopped breathing, or her heart could've—"

Val became abruptly light-headed. "That's enough, Jeff, whoa! I have to sit down—nauseous, nauseous!" But nevertheless, she urged me on, "So, you're in the procedure room and . . . ?"

"The doctor figures he's just numbed up my groin area with lido-caine, like he's done for my other angiograms. But all of a sudden my lips go numb, and then my tongue and my chin and my ears—can't feel 'em. And I'm dizzy and slow, and it's too much effort to breathe, so I call out, 'I can't feel my face—I think something's wrong here,' but the doctor and the resident and two nurses don't respond. I call out again, 'Hello! Something is very wrong!' And now they're scurrying— blood pressure monitor squeezing my arm, oxygen tubes under my nose—but no one's saying a word to me! I'm lying flat, right, because I've got an angiogram plug in my femoral artery, so I can't sit up and look anyone in the eye. I shout, 'Am I dying?' and still, no response— everyone's glued to the EKG monitor. And I realize, holy shit, it's get-ting harder to form words—like my mouth isn't working or something! So I force myself to get super calm and focused—'cause I'm thinking this might be the last thing I ever say—and I put it to them loud and clear: 'Someone—tell me right now what is happening here—because if you don't and I wind up dying on this angiogram table, I swear—*I am going to haunt every one of you*—and you'll never sleep again—you'll be in bed at night and hear chains dragging across your ceiling, and it will be the ghost of *me . . .*'"

Val gasped. "You didn't!"

"I sure did. And you know what? That doctor zoomed right over and said sorry—told me he'd shot the lidocaine straight into my vein by accident and was going to watch me very closely until my body absorbed it."

"That's the least he could do, the jerk. But, Ames, the *I'm going to haunt you*—ha! You must've freaked out everyone in that room—scared the hell out of them."

"I sure hope so. But Scott said it's out of line . . . and that it doesn't help in stressful situations when people are working on my body and I add extra pressure into the room. He's right."

"Yeah, but look—those people acted terribly. You felt like you were going to die—you could have died! And they just kept ignoring you when you called out to them. You were not your best polite self in there, okay, but I get why you said what you said. You were scared beyond comprehension and you wanted everyone around you to feel some of that terror for themselves."

She had put words to my motivation before I could make sense of it myself. Thanks to her husband's medical input, she appreciated the direness of an errant lidocaine injection. Val has also seen more than her fair share of alarming medical sights while caring for close family members who had battled serious illness over the years—including her father, her husband, and her son. But there was something else that heightened her empathy as well—a difference between Val and my other close friends (and even my husband) that allowed her to plunge beneath the surface and come up with exceptional insight into my reality, time and again: her sensitivity to the unreliability of appearances.

"That pharmacist probably took one look at you in your cute jeans and T-shirt, with your hair all nice and those terrific arm muscles you've got going on there—and she lost her bearings," Val says. "You're too thin"—she nudges the cashew bag toward me—"but you don't look sick, Ames. And that's a problem, because everyone around you, even medical people, forgets all you've been through. I mean—everyone even forgets the double mastectomy you had just a couple of months ago!"

"*You* don't forget."

"You're right. But I'm in a unique position. Think about it— after the lidocaine fiasco, we spoke on the phone, that's all. I was in Durham, so I couldn't meet you for coffee the next day, like maybe Lauren did. I didn't see you sitting across from me in your workout clothes, looking perfectly well when you told me that the doctor screwed up and shot lidocaine into your vein. No, I only got to *hear* you—that's all I ever get to do. I'm never thrown off by the way you look, so I have a whole different perspective on what a week is like in your body."

It's our evening phone calls that have made this possible. Val is my only friend who will notice just how many trips I've made to the hospital over a short time period. "You're *never* well," she'll note with sadness, whereas another friend may see me at the supermarket one afternoon and rave, "You look great!" As it turns out, an accurate perception of our friends' lives depends more on consistent, careful attention than geographic proximity. The many miles between Val and me—I recognize now more than ever—are a limitation that has actually broadened and deepened our friendship. We understand each other better when the life stories and emotions we share are stripped of momentary appearances. Saying *I see*—and meaning it—requires a commitment of more than just the eyes, and Val and I seem to have made this commitment. Our listening feels like honoring.

"Thank you, Val!" I blurt out, overwhelmed by a surge of emotion. The years of closeness between us feel desperately precious all of a sudden. How fortunate I am for this friendship—and for all the friendships that have shown up in the chair where Val sits today.

The things I love about these women flood my awareness now—Jill's constancy . . . Lauren's intuition . . . Joy's enthusiasm . . . Leja's determination . . . Jody's kindness . . . Val's insight . . . Is it a wonder we've grown so bravely and beautifully along the timeline together from twenty-five to fifty? Friends are powerful growers; they're the earth *and* the sun *and* the water. What—*what*—will I do without them when my heart can't wait for its replacement anymore and all goes dark?

"I'm so grateful for our friendship," I cry, reaching out my arms toward my dear friend Val. She receives an embrace meant for many.

We're still in a tight hug when Dr. Kobashigawa comes in with his trademark "Hello, hello." He shakes my hand and then Val's, and sits in the chair opposite us, frowning gently. "I heard what happened with our pharmacist, and I—I'd really like to apologize. I was supposed to talk with you first, but things don't always happen in the order they're meant to. I take responsibility." He closes his eyes in a long, sorrowful blink.

Val's face lights up with awe. She's not yet familiar with the compassionate Cedars way, having heard for almost thirty years about the gruff treatment I received at Columbia, where my transplant doctor spoke to me in surly sentences that neither began nor ended with a kind word or handshake.

Dr. Kobashigawa goes on to impress her with a candid explanation of why I will need a series of eculizumab treatments ("Your antibodies are still considerable") as well as why I should be aware but not afraid of the risks involved. "It has been used very successfully and safely in kidney recipients, and now we've got a grant from the National Institutes of Health for a trial with heart transplant patients at Cedars. I think you will tolerate the treatments well—it is considered chemotherapy, yes, but not the kind you're probably thinking of. Basically, eculizumab is a complement inhibitor and monoclonal antibody . . ."

Val's eyes go wide. "Huh?"

"That means the eculizumab will inhibit my body from binding complement so I'll be less likely to have an antibody-mediated rejection," I say. I'd made my way through enough of the eculizumab binder to understand and memorize the drug's basic mechanism.

"I have no doubt you understand, Amy." He gets up from his chair and says to Val, "Your friend here is pretty sharp."

"I know. I was her law school roommate!" She smiles dreamily at the back of the doctor's white coat on his way out. After he's cleared the door, she grabs her spray bottle and presses the button that powers its fan attachment. "*Aaaah . . .*"

"I'm going to apologize," I tell her.

"To Scott?"

"No, the pharmacist. First thing tomorrow morning."

"Good. And don't you think Scott also deserves—" She falls abruptly silent, leaning onto her elbow and dropping her chin into her hand. "Never mind. More cashews?"

From: Valerie Yablon
Subject: Just for you two
Date: April 22, 2014 at 7:36 PM
To: Lauren Steale, Joy Ceterra

The guard has surely changed; Joy, you are a tough act to follow. I have to say, Amy looks amazingly well. It's hard to believe from looking at her that anything is wrong.As for me, after two full days and nights without leaving this room, I am surprisingly fine. If I had to function in my real life I wouldn't be, but since I am focused only on Amy, little sleep is ok. I do feel rather helpless, though. Dr. K came this morning and acknowledged several times that Amy is very sick, saying he will keep his fingers crossed for a donor at the soonest—perhaps this weekend. Amy picked up on that and it made her feel very scared.Oh please let it be tonight, as she won't tolerate too many more days like today.She begged me to put a pillow over her head right before she drifted off to sleep a few minutes ago. And poor Scotty, he got the worst of it today.Leja returns tomorrow—a great help, for sure.

xo

IT'S THE THIRD and final night of Val's visit, and she's determined to do something about my complete lack of fresh air. The large picture window to the left of my bed doesn't open, and I'm not allowed to take the hospital elevator to the lobby and step outside—not even for two minutes—because, as Dr. Lunchbox explained, it would require accompaniment by a nurse *and* a doctor. "What if you had a cardiac episode?" he warned. "It's too big a risk."

"It's not exactly healthy for you to be cooped up in this room either," Val harrumphs, getting up from her chair. "I'm going to do something about it right now!" She perches on the windowsill and then stands up to inspect a smaller sliver of window that is set way up above the larger one. It turns out to be casement style, which suggests that a shift of its handle may pop it out sufficiently to allow a few inches of open space. "Aha! Watch this!" She tries again and again to crank it open. "Could they make this any harder!"

"It's probably against the rules, Val. And hey, you'd better speed it up before Justin gets in here. Medicine's at ten . . ."

"Grrr, arhh!" She strains, pushing and pulling, and then, *creak-thump*, it opens. "Good grief!" Val exhales, squatting down and descending the ledge shakily. She stands with her hands on her hips, catching her breath for a few seconds.

I laugh, applauding. "You know I love that *good grief* thing. I mean, who says that? Only you, Val. And only you would think to climb your crazy ass up there to open that window."

"Six weeks without a breath of fresh air? Yeah, I'm climbin', all right!" She waves me off with her hand. "I wanted to be sure to leave you with at least one concrete improvement before I go home tomorrow."

I guess she doesn't see the indelible marks of her presence as I do. Val certainly has made changes here, just as the others did before her. She has contributed a definite New Age sensibility. There's the lavender spray bottle, which she set upon my night table for a quick, calming aromatherapy *pssst* during pacemaker firings. Next to it sits a Tupperware container filled with sand from the Santa Monica shoreline—gathered and transported by Jody, who, after meeting Val for the first time two days ago and asking if there was anything she needed, found herself complicit in Val's holistic prescription that *sand play is so therapeutic!*

There's also the cautious, germophobic edge she brought on board. It started with the cheap bedroom slippers she'd purchased specifically for this trip, as Val wouldn't dare touch her feet to the presumably bacteria-ridden hospital floor. In the same vein, the cot's surface gave her the creeps due to the incalculable number of strangers who had slept on it; after cringing through her first night of sleep, she resorted to putting an air mattress on top of the cot, thereby creating a double-decker bed.

Truth be told: I'll be glad to see the double-decker sleeping arrangement disassembled after Val leaves; the rub of the air mattress against the plastic cot cover sounds like a giant balloon animal being made over and over again, all night long.

But I am also going to miss that squeak; it reassures me that it is Val specifically who's there in the darkness, ready to fly to my bed and nurture me through the pain like no one else. She has a different approach to laying hands—I don't know if it comes from the way she's mothered her two sons or if it's just her natural response to a demanding new circumstance. But her technique has turned out to be surprisingly affecting. Rather than sit beside me on the bed, she slides behind and stretches out her legs on either side, straddling me like a Lamaze birthing partner or a yoga teacher with very loose boundaries, saying, "Breathe, breathe."

It felt awkward at first—more so than Jill or Joy or Lauren sitting at my side, rubbing my feet or stroking my back. Even those moments felt uncomfortable at first because they broke through the quick hug-and-kiss boundaries we were used to. But after the second or third time that Val climbed boldly into position, I felt a complete enveloping. It was all-in and steadfast, and it relieved my concern that the sixth or tenth pacemaker firing might wear out her support.

And with Val sitting directly behind me, I could be spared the look of distress I'd seen on the faces of friends who'd preceded her. Val couldn't keep watch over the EKG monitor from where she sat, but she didn't care to; counting the seconds or testing my ability to predict the cessation of each painful wave was not her way. Val's approach had its own focus and daring—she grabbed on and held me steady through every second of trepidation like a skydiving guide in a tandem jump, landing me safely again and again.

She reaches into her suitcase now and pulls out a toiletry bag and hand towel. "Just use my bathroom—it's fine," I tell her. "I'll suspend Joy's rule since it's your last night here." I imagine that using the visitors' bathroom in the hallway has been a disgusting challenge for her.

"I accept!" She smiles and shuffles her slippers across the room.

A text pops up on my cell phone—*ting ting!*

"It's Casey. He says he's going to FaceTime me in a couple of minutes," I call out over the sound of running water.

Val pops her head out of the bathroom, toothbrush in mouth. "Good! Good!"

"I gotta doll myself up a little," I warn. I pull off my pajama top and replace it with a lilac shirt, then head to the bathroom to put on a little blush and fix my hair. "Pardon," I say, edging in on the mirror while Val flosses her teeth. "Can't let Casey see me looking sick."

"You don't look—" The FaceTime tones ring out.

"I hope you're right!" I retrieve my laptop from the bed and sit in Lauren's chair by the door so there won't be an EKG monitor in the background. I try to catch my breath before answering the call. "Hi, Case! What's up?"

We chat about his classes, his weekend plans, the weather in Ohio. I take care to smile and keep things light, and Casey follows my lead. We know no other way; he's been raised on normal appearances despite serious illness. I tell him Val is visiting and turn the laptop in her direction—"Wave to Casey, Val!"—and soon we wrap up with a quick "Miss you!" I feel a cry lump rising up in my throat, but I fend it off abruptly with a happy good-bye. "Oh, and Case," I add, "I'll be out of here pretty soon. The doctor says I'm at the top of the list now."

"That's great, Mom."

"And when school lets out in May, you can come and hang with Dad and me. I'm going to have to stay in LA for a couple of months after the surgery."

"Sounds good. Love you."

"Love *you*, Case. Bye."

Val makes a sad face at me, standing in her pajamas and puffing out her lower lip before climbing onto the double-stacked bed. "I miss him so much," I tell her, deflating after my strong-mom act. I change back into my pajama top.

Val sighs. "You take very good care of him."

"I can't, really, from this hospital bed."

"No. What I mean to say is that you spare Casey—a lot."

"Yeah, I do. I always have. And I'm not going to start clobbering him over the head with my illness *now*." I pull the string that hangs above my night table, and the lights go off. I settle under the covers while Val squeak-squeaks her way into a comfortable position. "Okay, then, good night, Val," I say.

"Good n— Hey, can I just point something out? You okay to stay awake a few minutes?" *Squeak-creak-squeak*—it sounds like maybe she's shifted onto her side to face me. But I can only see her vague silhouette in the greenish glow of the EKG monitor.

"Sure."

"So—you got *dolled up* for Casey's FaceTime call, right? But when Scott brought dinner here for us tonight, well, let's just say you didn't get so dolled up or spare him how sick you feel—just the opposite."

"It's too much effort to look good, especially at the end of the day. And I don't have to hide things from Scott."

"Don't you? Just a little bit? And this isn't just about how you look—I would guess that Scott doesn't really care if you put on nice clothes. But you could make an effort to watch out for his *feelings* sometimes, you know? Like with the pharmacist. You apologized to *her*. But with Scott, you dug in deeper."

"I wanted him to understand my position."

"I have to tell you, Ames . . . a little *less* understanding might do Scott some good. You can keep your thoughts to yourself sometimes and just spare him. You know? I don't mean to overstep . . ."

But Val has just taken a sizeable leap—straight into the center of my marriage—and I think it's no coincidence that she's waited until nighttime to do it. Here in the darkness, we've returned to our familiar place of unseeing, where honesty commands less daring. Husband talks are often limited to poking fun and sparking lighthearted commiseration (*He's standing in front of the refrigerator saying "I don't see the milk," and it's right there in front of him . . .*); when they do turn serious, taking the husband's side in a conversation with a friend—be it Val or anyone else—is almost never done.

But the rules of husband talk can be broken here in the hospital room. In the seclusion of this magical space with its long, long hours of privacy and its now-or-never sense of time, all limits in subject matter are off. Propriety shifts. Convention turns useless. Friends come to see quickly that the bright spot in the dark of this room—and what makes the best in each of us shine within it—is complete openness and honesty. Within these unusual walls, it is what we fail to say (or share, or admit, or raise) that will likely lead to regret—not the opposite.

Val is the latest to break through the unspoken friend boundaries. She'd only just shaken off the residual anxiety of a year of medical hardships—including the death of her father and a surgery for her husband—when my heart took a fast turn. And now Val is back in a hospital room without mobility, sleep, and fresh air, her short-lived sense of peace again interrupted. There isn't much for Val to gain in this visit—except time alone with me and, perhaps, coming away with a sense that she's made a positive difference that may continue on after she goes home. How can I be upset with her, then, for trying to leave her mark in any way she can? Veering into husband territory is not all that different from her insisting on cashews or lavender mist bottles or straddling back rubs. Val means to heal me.

"If you just spare him the littlest bit, it would be so appreciated. Believe me, I should know," she says, "because I'm on the other side of it with Jeff. I'm the caretaker. And sometimes, I get furious with him just for being sick—again."

For longer than I've had a heart transplant, Jeff has had colitis.

"I wouldn't ordinarily say this out loud, but I'm going to tell you anyway so maybe you can understand Scott a little better. I know, of course, that Jeff is the one who's suffering when his flare-ups strike, and I feel awful for him. I love him so very much, and I'm glad to be there for him every minute. But when his thoughts get revved up and he wants to tell me all the terrible things that could possibly happen to him in the future because of his condition, sometimes, I just wish he'd keep his fears to himself. Because there's nothing I can say to make things better. And I think that's how Scott feels. It's twenty-six years you've been sick. You exceeded your life expectancy by a crazy mile. Scott is scared enough of losing you without hearing every little thing that pops into your— Uh . . . I don't mean to say *little* thing. They're horrible things, and very real—for you *and* for Jeff."

"But we're supposed to keep them to ourselves."

"Not all of them. Just some. And any time you can take Scott's feelings into account, you know, smooth things over—like after you made the pharmacist cry—you should do it. You've been sick almost since the day he met you . . . The guy is *tired*. And I understand those feelings, of course . . ."

I had the chance to see Val's exhaustion firsthand a few years ago when Jeff wound up with a dangerous infection after a routine surgery. At the first sign of Val's readiness to accept my help, I flew to Durham and I found Jeff in a terribly weakened state; he needed Val's constant assistance as well as her tending to his IV antibiotics every few hours. She cared for him with diligence and grace until day's end, when she ran out of energy and abundant patience, wearied from medical detail as well as preparing breakfast, lunch, and then dinner according to his needs and expectations. We joined Jeff at the table and then sat in tense silence as he picked through his food and struggled in obvious pain through each bite. "Val, more water," he demanded with uncharacteristic abruptness, pointing to his empty glass.

She flushed crimson. "Do you think you could say please? Or, better still, could you just get up and get it yourself?"

Jeff could have managed both. But I understood how, in his arduous state of healing, he could be more focused on his own needs than on ways to give Val a small break. "I should have just gotten the water for him," she lamented later that night. I didn't know how to respond to her at first; I thought Jeff's tone was jarring—but also familiar. I'd heard the same in my own voice many times when frustration and agony won out over gentleness and considerateness.

"You're loving and wonderful to Jeff," I told her.

She's squeaking around on the double-decker bed now, and the light of a just-opened iPad illuminates her face for the first time tonight. She turns to look at me. "You gotta start sparing Scott a little. I saw it in his eyes, he's spent. And here's the last thing I'll say, and then you can go to sleep and I'll write this email: patience for a child is unlimited . . . but for a spouse, it's just not."

Val had great aim. Her words hit me right where she intended: smack in the center of my soft spot for her younger son, Sam, who, at two years old, underwent brain surgery. Her immense determination and maternal stamina not only nursed him through recovery from major surgery, but also has been a health-giving constant over the sixteen years since then, during which time Sam overcame obstacles to become a varsity athlete and scholar with acceptances to some of the best colleges in the country. Val and I spent many hours over the last few days talking through Sam's choices for next year and making comparative lists. What a joyous undertaking for us, and an attestation of Val's limitless devotion to Sam and his every need.

"You're exactly right," I say, turning on my side to face her. I feel thankful for this rare exchange with my friend. It's not marital advice that she has just given me; it is life wisdom of the sort I don't hear from other friends. Val is the only one in my inner circle who lives every day with the constant specter of medical problems in her home. Even though she's not sick herself—"How can I get sick when I have to take care of everyone else?" she has joked—Val's nearness to illness makes me feel joined to her. She has had to turn medical challenges into insight. She finds little peace in the passing of time. She understands the permanence of memories and the scary possibilities rooted in the medical histories of her husband and son. How could she not believe in the power of okra chips and coconut water and a single window cranked open a few inches? In her presence the last few days, I myself have been thinking about hummingbirds, and allowing my mind to mull over Ena's pronouncement that *God is everywhere*. If hopeful imagery takes the place of rational thought at times, that's fine with us. We're both just doing the best we can.

But now I have to start doing better.

I pull the string beside my bed and the light comes on. I shift myself into a sitting position and take a deep breath. "I don't know where to start with Scott," I admit. "There's so much I've done wrong."

"Well, just keep his feelings in mind and go from there. I'm sure there'll be plenty of chances for you to do things right."

"Yeah. Remember we used to say that when our boys were little?"

"What?"

"More chances to get it right. Like when Casey dropped his Popsicle in the park and he screamed his head off and wouldn't get out of his stroller and play—and these mothers are looking at me like, *Can't you control your kid?*—so I bought him another Popsicle just to shut him up? Bad lesson to teach him. Bad Mommy moment. And you told me, 'Don't sweat it—wait a few hours, and Casey will give you another chance to do it better.'"

"That's right! Oh, our boys gave us chances all day long."

"And that's why we were such great mothers!" I'm smiling now, but I feel my chest starting to tighten. The heaviness is setting into my arms and shoulders. "Val, sorry, I think the pain is starting . . ."

She dismounts from her perch at once—*SQUEAK!*—"I'm on my way . . ." In seconds, I feel her behind me, settled into position. "Scratch, tickle, or rub?" she asks, releasing a few pumps of lavender spray into the air.

The burning is already full force. "*Ow, ow*—tickle, I think."

"Okay, good. That's my signature move. It did the trick for Sam, you know, when they had to go back in about a week after his surgery to relieve the pressure. His head was so swollen, poor baby . . ."

They had to go back in?

How did I not know that?

Where was I during Sam's long hospitalization anyway? Casey was about four or five years old at the time, I guess; Scott could have helped out with his after-school care. I could have gotten on a plane and flown to help Val with anything she might need—picking up her other son at school, fixing meals for the family, maybe giving her a back rub at the end of the day.

But I didn't.

Come to think of it, I didn't even consider showing up to support my friend when her two-year-old son had surgery . . . on his brain.

I was an idiot.

"Should I scratch now?" Val asks. "This is a long pacing, huh? Just tell me if I should change it up." Another two pumps of lavender.

"Change—" I can't speak in full sentences once the pain gets this sharp. And since I've gotten pretty adept lately at holding back from wailing during pacemaker episodes, the room takes on a solemn, almost meditative silence in between Val's words and sprays.

Did I even call her when Sam was recovering? Did I send a fruit platter? No.

I was, what, thirty-three? I'd been close to death myself not too many years before; you'd think I would have known better. But I didn't. And back when we were twenty-five, Val didn't either. During the two months her law school roommate spent waiting for a donor heart at Columbia, I think she came to visit only once or maybe twice.

We were the closest of friends. But we were idiots.

Well, not anymore. Life, as it turns out, gave us many more chances to get better at friendship. Thousands of phone conversations later, we knew when to come running.

"Is it easing up at all?" she asks.

"A little . . . It should be over any second now." I know the timing all too well. "Please, Val . . . go on and head back to your cot . . . get some sleep while you can. You must be so tired. Sorry."

She maneuvers out from behind me. "Nah, I'm great. Really. I'm happy to pop up again and again if you need me. I've totally found the right way to do this—the straddling technique."

"Yeah, you totally have."

Look at that.

Look at us.

Doing it the right way.

Extraordinary.

I see it now: this second transplant has given Val and me the chance to return at fifty to the same context that overwhelmed us at twenty-five and thirty-three—and to do it right. It's like one of those movie plots where you get to go back to high school and live it all over again, this time with a wiser, stronger, better you inside. Near-death, it turns out, provides a ripe background for great life lessons. And each of my friends—Val included—has brought her unique qualities and insights to bear in boldest form, crossing boundaries and taking chances with honesty so that I might spend this hospital-room time in the way Scott had hoped I would—more thankful than bitter, more inspiring and inspired than just plain sad. The drama of illness was going to have its fated path for sure, but the story of how that path would teach and change all of us was ours to play out until—well—*The End.*

"Love you, Val," I say once the pain has subsided completely. "And yeah, I've got to ease up on Scott—give him a break wherever I can manage it. Thanks for that."

"That's so good to hear, Ames. Good night."

I reach up for the pull cord and give it a yank. The light goes off.

My silence after the pacemaker implantation was, Scott told me weeks ago, the last straw. I was not to let myself sink to that level of inconsiderateness and misconduct again. He made it clear that there could be no more.

No. More.

But then I ran out on Jill inexplicably on mud-mask night.

And I sent the pharmacist sobbing out the door.

And in between those episodes, there were about half a dozen other lashings out—as Scott saw them to be—where I acted like someone other than the Amy he knew and loved. On these occasions, I would lose all grace and kindness, and whirl a path of destruction through the room— with barbed responses, barked demands, and ornery musings that started with jabs like So, when I'm dead, and you're still alive . . .

The night before Val flew home to North Carolina, Scott took me in his arms. Val noticed us curled up on the bed together and took it as a signal to double-spritz lavender over our heads before she stepped into the hall to give us privacy.

"I've been trying to think of how I can help you hold on to yourself and not act in a way that hurts you and everyone around you," Scott began. "And I've also wanted to find out for myself how I can deal with it better— maybe talk with someone who's got expertise in medical crises."

He said a friend had connected him with a physician and professor at Harvard Medical School who was also the director of an ethics and palliative care department. Scott had spoken with the guy just that afternoon—giving him a comprehensive overview of me and how I'd fared all these years, my medical history, the vasculopathy and pacemaker pain, and the inverted hourglass that was fast draining down on my heart time. He also described the inscrutable lapses in my behavior.

"And, you know," Scott said softly to me, "I thought he would give me a little . . . uh, support. Some understanding of how difficult it is to stand aside when anger and fear and frustration consume you and, well, make you act like . . ."

"A raving lunatic?" I kidded.

Scott smiled, pulling me in tighter. "Sort of, yeah."

He told the professor that he'd tried and tried, but just couldn't understand how his wife could turn so hurtful and belligerent at moments. "If I were sick and dying," he stated decisively to this professor, "I wouldn't do that."

The professor answered at once, "You don't have any idea what you would or would not do. No one can know until they're in it. Don't kid yourself."

Flat out.

I turned my head to look at Scott—his face was wide-eyed wonderment. The words struck him still.

"The guy had absolutely no empathy for me," he admitted. "And certainly no sympathy. Not even praise for all the patience I've shown you. He just put me in my place, all right. 'You don't have any idea.' And I thought— huh, whoa—he's right."

I brought my hand to the side of Scott's face, meeting his gaze with tears. "Thank you, my love."

9

---

ll rightie then—how 'bout now I show you the little surprisey-poo I've brought with me?" After a morning of mostly solemn talk we've hit a lull, and Jill decides at once to shift the mood by taking her voice up an octave and laying on the silly, sarcastic edge that is our nonsense way. "I'm so ex-*cccited!*" she adds, going even higher in tone while pulling her suitcase from under the cot. "*Surprisey-poo-poo!*" she trills again.

I play along, matching my intonation to hers. "Is it . . . *bigger than a bread box?*"

"Well . . . it's definitely funnier, I'll tell you that." She unzips a compartment and retrieves a plastic bag.

"Ah, so it's *funny*—hmm. I was thinking it might be a new heart you've got in there."

"No, sorry, but it does have to do with something that goes thumpity-thump, if you know what I mean, and I *know* you do!" She flashes me a twisted smile from where she's kneeling on the ground, "I'm referring to *love*, of course—try to keep it clean, you perv—"

"*You're* the perv."

"I know you are but—"

"What am *I*?"

We've become eleven years old again, total goofballs, and I'm feeling a lot lighter for it. Good thing it's just Jill and me in here, so that we can let loose. Jody has already come and gone for the day, and Leja isn't due to arrive for another few minutes. We wouldn't dare indulge in this ridiculous banter in their presence.

Jill sits down in a chair with the plastic bag on her lap. "Now, close your eyes. I've got something to read to you."

"All right." I quickly close them, but Jill delays with deliberate pause.

"*Ahem, ahem*"—she means this to be a dramatic reading. "I'm going to skip right to the good part, *ahem*—" There's a rustling of pages. She goes high pitch again:

They sit at their usual table in the back. The restaurant is dimly lighted and warm, and their hands are sweating because they are holding hands and they are always afraid someone might see. "Barry, there is something I have to tell you . . ."

My eyes pop open. "You still have a copy!"

"Not just a copy—the original! Get a load of this . . ." She shuffles the collection of pages and turns the top one toward me. "I think this is your cover art, right?"

"I can't believe it—yes!" The colored-pencil sketch I made in the sixth grade stares back at me, faded out by time, but clear enough to decipher the three red hearts I drew inside a large blue triangle, as well as the title of Jill's invention—*Triangle of Love*. I reach out for the makeshift book. "Let me see that!" It has been almost forty years since I held it in my hands.

"You're gonna *laugh*!"

I begin flipping through the pages. "Barry! Caroline! *Ha-ha* . . . talk about pushing the envelope!" Our sixth grade teacher's first name was Larry, and the teaching assistant in our classroom was Carol. I remember how it made us feel to write something so provocative; aiming our sexy story at two adults in our everyday life was, we thought, ingenious and a sure mark of our maturity.

"Take your time—read all the way through," Jill advises. "Then we'll talk. I've got to call the office anyway." She reaches for her laptop.

"'*Triangle of Love*, by Amy and Jill,'" I read aloud, turning the page. "'Dedicated to everyone who falls in love.' Oh please! What was wrong with us?"

"You don't know the half of it. Read on . . ."

Leja walks in just then and flops immediately into Lauren's chair near the door, flushed and trembling. "I see just now something so sad!" She thumps her open palm against her chest, catching her breath before more words spill out. "In the waiting room! A family! Seven or ten of these people, they kneel on the floor to praying. I stop and I look—*for who is it they pray?* And I talk with one of them. Oh, this is a terrible . . ." She brings her fist to her mouth and shuts her eyes tight.

Jill raises her eyebrows at me, curious but not surprised. She has known Leja for as long as I have and is plenty familiar with the intensity of her emotions. I hold up my hand to say, *Give her a few seconds . . .*

Leja shoots up from her chair and begins to pace. "The woman, she is thirty, and she is wait for a heart transplant in the intensive care. Husband, children, brother, cousins, kids—all in the waiting room . . ." She continues on, interspersing the story with words like *antibodies* and *total artificial heart* and *Swan-Ganz catheter*. I am impressed with Leja's knowledge, and the careful, exacting attention she pays to all she encounters here at the hospital, in spite of being overwhelmed by it. "So will be very long time before she can get heart. She has many, many antibodies like you do, but she can't be 1A because her kidneys, they do not work. Her creatinine is more than *three*, her husband tells to me."

Leja even understands creatinine blood levels as a measure of kidney function. She's been following my levels each day, after all—listening intently when Dr. Kobashigawa reassures me that my kidneys are doing remarkably well under the circumstances, and then repeating his words back to me later on when I imagine that my bloated feet mean kidney doom. Using real medicine as a resource is a marked change from the naïve and superstitious Leja, who, for as long as I've known her, has believed that cold drinks are actually the cause of the common cold. These two months in a hospital room have taken her medical acumen far beyond the Croatian old wives' tales that had been her prior source of reference.

But just about everyone on Six South is sick enough to warrant ICU stays and hallway prayers from family members, and Leja knows this. "They'll probably give her dialysis to support her kidneys, and she'll be back on the list soon," I reassure her.

"Yes, they can do . . . But her family, they are so poor and they can't to afford sleep in a hotel room in LA, so they must to live in the waiting room! They tell me they do not have a shower in so many days. They also do not have food enough . . ."

Leja explains that the extended family has rotated week to week in a vigil for this relative, who has been hospitalized for over two months now. They all live in northernmost California—about a seven-hour drive from Cedars—so they can't make the trip daily. They are thankful not to be chased out of the waiting room after hours. "The security guards who walk in the night, I think they are pretend not to see this family sleeping there, could be."

She's probably right. I've gotten wind of out-of-towners and their families being handled with sensitivity by Justin, Lachalle, and other staff who tend to the sixth floor. It seems a significant percentage of pretransplant patients come here from distant states or even foreign countries, having been sent by their local cardiologists because of Cedars's unique specialization in the most complex challenges—including dangerous antibodies like mine. Previous transplantation is not the only cause of troublesome antibodies; there are other patient groups who suffer this complication as well, including those who have had blood transfusions and women who are highly sensitized from pregnancies.

During my heart transplant orientation when first arriving at Cedars, I talked with a few of these relocated pretransplant patients who, like me, followed their doctors' urging and headed to LA. Of course, there was a good deal of commiseration about the financial burden of living in LA for an indefinite period of time. Scott and I have been extremely fortunate in this regard: Scott has been able to continue to work at his job via Skype and conference calls. But many patients I've met have had to ask for donations from their communities, Internet crowd-sourcing sites, or Facebook to help finance their long local stays. A couple of them said they might have to sacrifice college tuition for their children to pull this off. And now Leja has discovered the direst situation yet: a family contending with circumstances that has them sleeping in the waiting room for months at a time.

I tell Leja that we need to think about how we might be able to help this family. "Maybe Scott can invite them to the bungalow so they can all take a shower. Or maybe we can buy some sandwiches for lunch tomorrow. I don't know—it seems too small, but we should do something . . ."

"*Yes!* We must to do *something*! I will go tell to Scott now, okay? Then I must to leave for the airport." Leja was scheduled to fly home that afternoon to see her daughter. "I am sorry, Jill, that I cannot give you break."

"I don't need one," Jill says. "You need to get home for a few days of rest."

"No! I am not tired! It is okay to me!" She sweeps through the room with purpose, picking up bits of paper from the floor, tidying my night table, and refolding the throw blanket at the foot of my bed. "You have dirty laundry I can to take to bungalow!" she insists. (I don't, really, but I understand that concrete tasks calm Leja's nerves.) She opens my closet and holds up various clothing items, sniffing and inspecting. "This jeans? This shirt?"

"Take both, sure, great. Thank you, Leja."

She stuffs them into a plastic bag. "I go now and I talk with Scott when his business call is end. Bye!" She spins out the door, and the walls seem to exhale with relief.

"A woman on a mission—jeez, it's exhausting," Jill says.

"That's Leja."

"All that emotion—"

"The family in the hallway must've pushed her over the edge. She's seeing all kinds of sad things here. We all are. I mean, have you noticed there's a code blue announcement on the loudspeaker every few hours? It's a death knell. It means heart attack or breathing failure. The sights and sounds of this place can leave your emotions super raw if you let them. So"—I pick up the booklet I placed aside when Leja raced in— "let's get back to the fun stuff."

"Perfect," Jill says, reopening her laptop. "Tell me when you're done reading."

I settle into the pages again . . .

Her hair is long and straight and his is short and there is a small bald spot that should not be there because he is only thirty. She is taller than he is when she wears her platform shoes, so on this day she picks low heels . . .

Jill interrupts, "Hey, Ames—do you think it's allowed? Sleeping or praying or whatever in the waiting room overnight—you think the hospital is okay with that?"

I shrug. "Sometimes when a patient's condition is so precarious, family visitation rules get stretched really wide—it happened to me at Columbia. And the woman who's in the ICU here . . . if she's got failing kidneys *and* high antibodies, they've got to keep the family close, right? Her chances of survival are slim, sad to say it, and I don't mean to be a pessimist, but . . ."

"I get it. That article you sent me explained things—it's all pretty grim stuff." She bites down, and her lower lip disappears beneath her front teeth.

So Jill read it after all . . .

The article—a study published in a prominent medical journal—set out gloomy data on heart transplant mortality (especially retransplants), making clear that even if a patient lives to receive a retransplant, he or she may not survive very long after. Antibody-mediated destruction of the donor heart is the most serious threat to longevity in cases like mine, followed second by the high risk of immunosuppressant-related cancer (a risk that increases exponentially with accumulated years on transplant medications). If first-transplant lifespans tend to max out around ten years, second ones could be half that.

It would take guts to read past the first few lines of bad news like this. And since Jill didn't comment after receiving my email last week, I've had to wonder if maybe she cast it aside.

I wouldn't have blamed her if she did, considering that the previous article I'd sent her had forced the words *assisted suicide* in front of her eyes. But that mistake—as I now understand it to be—happened over a month ago, at a time when I felt I had to cry out in order to be understood. It was also before I'd come to carry in my mind (with stomach-churning guilt) the hurt and disappointment conveyed by Jill's silence the night I returned from my hallway sit-out. Seeing friends' reactions to my slipups in real time and close proximity these last few weeks has inspired me to try to do better. With every hand that strokes my back, and glance that meets mine with compassion, and voice that assures me, *I'm here for you, Amy,* I've felt myself moving further and further away from the impulse to hoist my *See me!* flag. Instead, I find myself considering more deeply the women around me, and learning from them by example: just as I am under their watchful care, they deserve to be under mine as well.

So, while I knew this journal article contained bad news that would no doubt be upsetting to Jill, I sent it nevertheless—because my true and deep motivation this time was to share the hard facts, not brandish them. The data-based reality was something we could understand together. Carry the weight of together. Perhaps cry about together.

"Thanks for reading it—I thought you might not want to . . ." I admit to Jill now. "It's tough stuff to swallow, I know."

"You're not kidding." Jill drops her head and shakes it slowly. "That ICU girl and her family don't know what they're up against. It's what *you're* up against, Ames." She lifts her sorrowful eyes. "There's no chance of a perfect ending here."

"Well, there's a chance at *life*—for how long, I don't know. But maybe the antibody treatments will make a difference." I pause, struck by how unusual it is that I—rather than one of my friends—am the one pointing out a bright spot in the dark now. "I've got to keep hope alive, or something like that, right? That's what a nurse at Columbia said to me once when I was hospitalized with an infection a few months after my first transplant—she actually scolded me: 'You *must* have hope! Always hope!' And I said, 'Why?' And you know what? She didn't have an answer—just 'You *must*!' It meant nothing to me at twenty-five, and I'm not sure it does now."

"Yeah, hope is a nice concept, but in practice it seems kind of . . . powerless."

"Which is why I've been thinking more about what another Columbia nurse said—she was the one who'd been with me for a bunch of heart biopsies and angiograms. She must have heard that I came out to Cedars for a transplant and got my cell number somehow. So, she called the other day and told me the cath lab staff was praying for me, and I said, 'Thank you, Margaret, but you know, there are so many people praying, all different faiths, some without any faith at all. Which god, then, is going to hear the prayer? It'll get too confusing.'"

"Yeah, yeah. It's like, why should a god listen to it if he knows there might be another god working on it already?"

"That's the idea. But the nurse, she told me, 'Don't worry because all these praying voices, see—they're *storming the universe!*'" I lift my hands into the air and wiggle my fingers for effect. "And that's when miracles happen. Or so she says."

"Whoa!" Jill grips the arms of her chair. *"Storming the universe . . ."* Her voice goes high pitch. "I *love* that!"

"Me too. Me too." I lift the paper book from my lap again. "Now, back to our masterpiece . . ."

A LITTLE WHILE later, Robin surprises us with an early arrival. She didn't send a text from the airport like the visiting friends who'd come before her. *Why impose?* was probably Robin's thinking. She even refused to give Scott her flight information for fear that he would insist on picking her up at the airport. Robin wouldn't want to be anticipated or fussed over this way—not one bit. For as long as I've known her, she's been intent on making her needs invisible and has done a steady job of it. I assured Scott, "You've got to let Robin just do her thing."

Robin's thing amounts to pretty much this: sharp mind, fierce independence, and remarkably productive chaos. She careens into my room with shopping bags lining her arms, a purse over one shoulder and a tote bag over the other, managing somehow to pull a loose-wheeled suitcase behind her.

"Amyyyyy . . ." she tolls, low and long like a foghorn. Her face is a combination of measured joy and all-out pathos—a proportional mix that fits well in this setting. But I've seen Robin bring this same expression to other circumstances in the past, including exam week during our first year of law school, when the dorm suite she shared with Val and me became a den of toil and tension. The three of us would emerge from our individual rooms, equally bleary-eyed from study, but then Robin would act is if only Val and I were inundated with pages and pages of law cases to review. She would ask how we were doing, and even if we said "Great!" she'd twist her face into a smile-frown, urging, "Well—you hang in there!"

Val and I would look at each other: *We* should hang in there?

It didn't make sense. Robin was just as stressed for time as we were, but she never showed it. It wasn't until second semester that the mechanism of her behavior became clear: Robin was hell-bent on being the absolute lowest maintenance, and this required her to take on a sort of *I'm okay—you're not okay* disposition. Once I figured this out, I started saying things in return like, "Well, *you* hang in there too!"—but this was short-lived because I realized that her intent had actually been kindness all along. As the months raced toward year-end grades and the cutthroat competition that would determine *Law Review* picks and plum summer jobs, I felt increasingly thankful to come home each day to the sympathies and empathies Robin strewed around our dorm room like flower petals.

And so, today, the concerned tone of her greeting is an echo from the past that stirs my appreciation. "Robin, you're here! Yay!" I cheer. She lurches toward me, still encumbered by baggage. "Wait, put down your stuff first," I say, helping her peel off some of the load.

Jill calls out from a chair on other side of the room, "Hi, Robin!"

"Jill, good to see you! Let me just hug Amy for a sec, then I'll come over there." She drops the last of her bags and reaches out to me, "Amyyyy! Ohhhh!" Then Jill gets hers, "Jiiiill! Ohhhh!"

They embrace like old friends, but they're only thinly acquainted. "When was the last time you guys saw each other? At my wedding?" I ask.

"Nah—I think it was at Scott's fiftieth birthday thing at your house," Robin says. "So, how've you been, Jill?"

"Good! Good! And, you?"

"Great. Great . . ."

Silence.

Long silence.

Jill stretches her arms toward the ceiling and yawns—sort of. Robin looks down at the array of shopping bags on the floor, mulling.

Uh-oh.

I didn't think about it until now, but this double-visitor arrangement may wind up being awkward. Jill and Robin sure aren't here to catch up on each other's lives; they're here to spend what may be our last hours together, giving their all to our conversations and to the latest task outlined by the spreadsheet friend who wrote the last email. But I have only one back that needs scratching. One minifridge from which to pull a bottle of cold water. And one small space beside my bed, which happens to be big enough to hold only one cot comfortably. But even more than logistics, the introduction of a third friend's voice into the mix of conversation will likely drain some of the content. I talk with Jill differently than I do Robin. Jill and I will have to hold back on our private banter—not only because it's unintelligible to others, but also because it would exhibit our extraordinary closeness in a way that might make my friendship with Robin seem less dear. At the same time, the intense, almost scholarly way that Robin and I deconstruct personal issues in our conversations might leave Jill feeling adrift on the surface of things.

This arrangement wasn't my idea. It was Joy's. And Lauren's. And, in most active part, Jill's. Apparently, there was a caucus among these three—or so Joy told me when she was here last—and they decided to depart from the one-friend-at-a-time format (which figured in Jody and Leja as daytime adjuncts) and pair Jill with Robin, "because, well, your pacing is getting worse and worse, and you have to feel that you can rely completely on the person who's there with you at night," Joy insisted. This meant bringing back an experienced spreadsheet friend who'd already visited and making her Robin's copilot.

I didn't argue. The nighttime pacing episodes were coming at shorter intervals now, and the duration of each one barely left me minutes to gather myself before the next. And although the group emails provided Robin with the basic protocol for back scratching and foot rubbing through my pain, it was the personal element added by each visiting friend, really, that worked the caring magic that brought relief—not just from physical anguish, but from the sadness and fear and despair that worsened with each passing day. Jill's flair was humor and unfailing empathy. Lauren's was depth of thought. Joy's was full-on engagement. Val's was compassion. Though there were numerous possibilities, I wasn't sure yet what Robin's flair would be.

Robin has always been a whirling wonder. From law school to marriage to motherhood to work life, she's seemed a bit slapdash at times—and yet has managed to produce impressive results that dazzle me. She has three gleaming, successful children and a happy husband on top of an attention-devouring and hour-consuming high-level VP/general counsel position at a major pharmaceutical company. Somehow she still manages to bring full energy to all the varsity ice hockey games, back-to-school nights, birthday parties, and evening walks with the dog. Robin races from one vital task to the next, improvising brilliantly, never in obvious frenzy but often with wide, darting eyes that are a cross between high energy and the panic of an unconquerable to-do list. (She conquers it every time, though.)

Robin throws herself into the task at hand now, seizing a plastic shopping bag from the floor and thrusting it toward me. "Here. I brought you a bunch of stuff. Take a look . . ."

I retrieve a few small items from inside the bag—lip gloss, a tube of body cream, a sample-size perfume vial, and a jar of face moisturizer. "Oh, wow, so thoughtful of you . . ." I say, reaching in for more, and then more; the bottles and tubes and jars keep on coming. "Look at all this!"

"Yeah—I just grabbed it all from my drawer. It's stuff from I don't know when. Gifts, samples from cosmetic counters . . ." She points to two green jars on my lap. "I think those were gifts for my twentieth wedding anniversary . . ."

That was five years ago. I smile and make a note to self: *Toss green jars.*

Robin picks up a tube, screws off the cap, and sniffs. "This one's nice." She passes it under my nose.

"Pretty!" I say, and then take hold and try to empty a bit onto the back of my hand—*squeeze, squeeze, squeeze*—but nothing comes out.

Robin notices my confusion. "Yeah, I have no idea, sorry. You know me—I was working late every night this week, and then I rushed this morning to make my flight . . ."

"No problem! There's plenty of good stuff to choose from in here . . ." I look down at the random accumulation in my lap, considering how the potential for germs is fairly high. When I look up again, Robin is holding a light blue shopping bag in front of my face. "Now what's *this*?" I recognize the name of the store printed in white.

"Open it."

Cotton pajama bottoms in a cool gray leopard-print, plus a tank top and silky soft robe—beautiful, stylish, thoughtful, and brand-new! I knew how difficult it must have been for Robin to take the time from her frenzied work/home life to get herself to a fancy little boutique just to pick out some sleepwear.

"Where'd you get *that*?" Even high-styled Jill is intrigued. She reaches for the robe and swoons over its buttery softness.

"There's a little place in Larchmont . . ."

"Is it that bra store, or . . ."

"No, that's across the street. It's actually a gift store that's . . ."

Off they go, chatting about suburban shopping spots and how the color gray is such an adorable choice for leopard print.

I lie back against the bed pillows and smile.

SCOTT HAS TAKEN Jill and Robin to lunch. It's another California blue-sky day and I insisted that they all get out and enjoy a bit. "Food tastes better outside hospital walls—and I'm *fine*, so please, go breathe some air."

"I can have lunch here with you and the girls can go by themselves," Scott offered. But I declined. So now I'm here alone—which feels odd because I've had constant company for so many weeks now. "We'll be back in half an hour, just half an hour," Scott assured me.

I told him to take his time. "Nothing's going on. I think I'll read."

But I find myself just sitting in the stillness, observing. There's so much purple in here now, and bright green. Peace signs and tie-dyes and horizontal strips of chalkboard (*Friends on duty: Jill and Robin*, it reads today). Busy walls, busy windows, busy bed pillows. Even in the silence, I sense the clamor of it. I close my eyes and listen to the street sounds through the crack of open window that was Val's parting gift.

The phone rings. Not my cell, but the old-fashioned push-button hospital phone that sits on my night table.

"Hello?"

"Hi, Amy, it's Emily . . ." I lose my breath—Emily is the transplant coordinator who manages donor heart offers for Cedars patients. "We might . . . have a heart for you . . ." She's speaking so carefully, so damn slowly. ". . . but . . ."

Ah, the glitch: There's another patient who is first in line for this heart, Emily tells me. I'm the fallback. More specifically, UNOS, the organization that maintains the national transplant waiting lists as well as the computer program that determines the appropriate heart recipient (i.e., the longest-waiting, sickest patient who is a blood-type and antibody match in the region, usually), has me at number two.

"We need to prepare you as if this is a go," Emily says. "'Cause sometimes, the heart winds up being too big or too small for the first on the list, and it goes to the second. Or a bunch of other things can happen. So don't eat anything—you've got to have an empty belly if there's a surgery. And I'm going to send someone from the team to take lots of blood for the cross-match, okay? So you just sit tight. I'm excited for you, Amy!"

"Could this really be it?" I ask, feeling my breath begin to quicken.

"It could. I've seen it happen before."

"Thank you, Emily! Thank you!" I hang up the phone.

I'm panting, and my excitement mixes with awe and wonder. The one time I'm alone in the room—it's only been about ten minutes since Scott and the girls left—I get a heart offer!

Well, almost an offer.

I call Scott's cell. He answers and I burst into tears. "Emily called!

I might have a heart! Come back!" Minutes later, Scott, Jill, and Robin rush through my doorway, out of breath from running. They dive onto my bed, tug at my arms with excitement. "What did you hear? Start at the beginning . . . word for word!"

The joyous roughhousing has me giggling, but I gather myself in spite of it so I can tell them, precisely, that I am second in line. "There's someone sicker than I am," I explain, "so they get it first." But the fact that I'm being prepped for surgery means that there's a real chance that the heart might wind up mine. The blood cross-match, I tell them, is even more encouraging. This means that my blood will be drawn here at Cedars and then transported to the donor hospital, "so that my blood can be mixed with the donor's to see if we sort of get along quietly, or if there's a bad reaction."

"Oh my God!" Jill beams. "This could really happen!"

"Yeah, and I'm going to have to shower with this special antibacterial soap—oh, and I'm going to want to wash my hair and make it nice since I won't be washing it for a week after surgery, probably . . ."

Scott is pacing with excitement. Robin is bouncing in her chair. Jill takes out her cell phone and asks, "Can I text the girls?"

"Um . . . I don't know, maybe not just yet," Scott says. "We don't know if this is really happening."

"Well, the prep is really happening," I say. "We should just tell them what the situation is, right? Scott, will you call my parents, please, and I'll call—"

"Hi there, everybody!" Lachalle walks in with a squeeze bottle in hand, smiling bright. "I heard you're number two. This could be your night—how about that now, how about that? So, you need to shower with this special soap—hair, body, everything."

"Can she use conditioner too?" Jill asks.

"Ha-ha, yeah, I think that would be all right."

"I want to be beautiful when I get my new heart!" I bubble. This is the happiest day—well, really the only happy day—in my hospital room so far.

"I like the attitude you've got there!" Lachalle says. "You go ahead and shower because they're coming to take your blood soon—ah, wait, here they are now . . ." She steps aside to make room for two very serious-looking nurses whom I've never seen before.

One of them has a harsh European accent. "We must hurry-hurry," she tells me, while the other nurse secures a strap around my upper arm. One, two, three—the needle is in and my blood begins to flow into what seems like endless vials. I look away from the sight, but I can hear the click-clack of blood tubes as they fill and get traded out for the next. The hurry-hurry nurse huffs while glancing nervously at her watch, "The helicopter, it is waiting on the roof. I will run there with this blood when we are done."

"Helicopter?" I say.

"To take your blood to the hospital where the donor is. For cross-match. Must get it there very, very quick."

"Where's the hospital?"

"Can I tell her?" she asks the kinder nurse who's drawing my blood.

"Yes."

"San Diego."

A few hours' drive would take too long, apparently.

Click-clack-click-clack-click-clack—the nurse gathers the tubes before the other nurse has pulled the needle from my arm. "I go now!" she announces, and runs from the room with a plastic bag filled to the brim.

"That was my favorite blood draw ever!" I joke. Everyone laughs. "Shower time!"

"Want me to help?" Jill asks.

"Sure, thanks." I start pulling off EKG leads from my chest.

"Let me help with the ones in the back," Robin says, taking the initiative and reaching under my T-shirt in search of them.

Just then, there's a loud whirring noise from outside. Scott, who's closest to the window and talking into his cell phone, points excitedly at the sky. Robin, Jill, and I crowd around him to get a look—it's a helicopter lifting off Cedars's roof.

"There goes my blood!"

"That's crazy! They were in here one minute ago!" Jill gawks.

"A-mazing!" Robin gushes.

We all come together in a big hug, surrounded by the sound of hope taking to the sky.

Minutes later, I toddle cheerfully to the bathroom for my antibacterial shower. I tell Jill I'll leave the door open and call her if I need help washing my hair. "All right, I'll do some push-ups and bicep curls to get ready for that—no kidding! Has anyone got a Red Bull?" She makes a he-man pose, flexing her muscles.

I'm going to try and do this myself this time, I decide, stepping into the shower. My strategy is to wash my hair first, before I get too weak. But within seconds under the hot water, I need to sit down on the shower bench. And after just a few rubs of shampoo against the surface of my hair—"Jill!" She pops into the bathroom at once. "I need help. Sorry," I tell her.

"Don't be silly." She takes the handheld shower attachment from me and starts to rinse out my hair, not realizing that I haven't fully shampooed it yet.

When I drop my chin to my chest, my eyes fall upon my grossly swollen feet, which are now dark blue, my distended belly, the transplant scar that runs from just above my navel to the base of my collarbone, and my still-fresh mastectomy sutures and tiny breast implants. As my eyes take in my own naked body, I'm suddenly feeling frantic and desperate to cover up, cover up! Everything is exposed. Not merely my surgical scars and my aging skin and my unshaven legs . . . but, rather, my . . . misfortune. I feel my body go rigid as she continues to rinse my hair. How excruciatingly self-conscious I am of its full-frontal view right this moment—*I don't want Jill to see, I don't want her to see.*

I take a deep breath and try to calm myself with a silent question: *Would I feel this way if Jill were my sister?*

Yes—because it's not so much embarrassment that makes me want to run for towel cover. It's more the naked exhibition of my nearness to death. From head to toe, there's no hiding the clear markings of what's ugly about heart transplants: they don't last as long as we hope they do, and if their years don't kill you with vasculopathy, their required medicines will slay you with cancer.

And here's Jill, my tireless friend who's working so hard—*Look at her with those dark circles under her eyes, so worn down by the days and nights in this hospital room.* She's doing all this to help me get to transplant number two? What a sad and ridiculous enterprise. Even if I am fortunate enough to receive a matching donor heart, the question will remain: Was it worth the toil of all of us? If my friends come to see that retransplant returns me to the precarious, ill state of health that characterized my last twenty-five years—or worse—will we all agree that this is too thin a victory, given the intensity of our effort?

These questions do not occur to Jill right now, I'm sure, no matter her exhaustion. It's so easy to get lost in the chase when the goal is life itself. It blinds you to the quality of that life.

"Are you all right?" she asks, noticing my sudden sadness.

"Soap in my eyes . . ."

"Oh, sorry about that. Here's a dry washcloth . . ." I dab my face and pop open the squeeze bottle of antibacterial body wash. "This could be the last shower you take with this heart—how about *that*?"

"How *about* that," I say.

AFTER A STRESSFUL evening with no news about the San Diego heart, Jill pushes her cot to the wall across the room, just beneath the giant collage of selfies, while Robin wedges hers between my bed and the window. They've got their laptops out now—Jill writes the nightly email and Robin does some work. I sit quietly, feeling especially cleaned up after my sudsy shower and all the beautification that followed. Jill and Robin sat me in a chair and blow-dried my hair, leaving it surgery-ready and prettier than it has been in weeks. Then they took time picking out which pajamas would bring us luck tonight (landing upon the pink, fine cotton ones that Lauren brought me but I haven't worn yet), and plucking stray hairs from my eyebrows. Jill filed my nails and Robin rubbed cream into the bottoms of my feet—primping and coiffing every possible part of me as if I'd been granted an audience before the wonderful Wizard of Oz. But it's almost eleven o'clock now, and our excitement is dissolving fast. "It shouldn't be taking this long," I say.

Robin closes her laptop and reaches out to me. Her cot is close by, and it feels like we're sharing a queen-size bed. "You're probably right. But it's not over until it's over." We hold hands and sit in silence for a few minutes.

The phone on my night table rings.

"Hello?"

It's Emily. She tells me things aren't looking good, but there's still a chance because there is no indication on the computer program that the first patient actually took the heart. The offer, then, is still considered open until UNOS marks it as *offer accepted.* "So why don't you go ahead and eat something if you want, because even if the heart winds up being yours, the surgery won't be until morning and that's plenty of time for your stomach to empty."

I take this as a bad sign. I know enough about surgeries to know that chances are never taken with food ingestion. "Emily, do you really think I've got a shot at this heart at this point?"

"I'll be honest with you, it is very strange that in ten hours there is not an updated status on the computer. You almost have to assume it's a glitch and the first patient on the list accepted the heart offer."

"What should I be thinking, then?"

"Sweetie, I think you should have some dinner—you must be really hungry. Order in a pizza, okay? Or maybe the nurse can bring you some apple sauce and graham crackers."

"Thanks, Emily." I hang up crying. Jill and Robin rush over and sit beside me on the bed. Each one of them takes a hand.

It's okay . . .

It wasn't your time . . .

It'll happen for you soon . . .

You'll be number one for the next heart . . .

I fall back against the bed pillows. "Robin, can you please get me a different pair of pajamas. These feel too happy."

"Yes, of course."

Everyone is wiping away tears. The room sinks to a new low of despair. "I just want to go to sleep and not wake up," I say, slipping the replacement pajama shirt over my head. Robin and Jill glance at each other. No response. "Never mind the pants," I tell Robin. "I don't have energy for them. I'm going to bed, ladies. This is just too damn sad."

Robin and Jill scurry back to their cots—*All right . . . good night, then . . . we're here for you when you need us . . . and we'll turn off the lights now . . . no more computers . . . let's all get some sleep . . . tough day . . .*

I hear Jill settling under the covers and Robin fluffing her pillow before lying down. They don't need to coordinate anything because earlier today they worked out an arrangement for tending to my nightlong pacemaker firings. Jill wanted to alternate, but Robin insisted that she take over since Jill had already racked up a few sleepless nights here. But I'm thinking I may not need either Jill or Robin tonight, since I expect I'll be wide-awake, racked with frustration and grief—and if I don't let my body relax and slip into sleep, there's a chance my pulse won't drop and my pacemaker won't fire.

Yeah, I think I'll just stay up all night, damn it . . .

After a few minutes, Robin's arm shoots up and then lands on my bed. "You asleep?" she whispers.

I turn on my right side to face her. "No. Too upset," I whisper back.

Robin slides to the edge of her cot so we can talk quietly without waking Jill. "I'm so angry about what happened today," she tells me. "I think it's cruel—to get your hopes up like that and then crash them to the ground. It's horrible."

"It's part of the transplant process . . ."

"It's inhuman! You're waiting and waiting, and they tell you, *Yeah, maybe we're going to save your life tonight*—and then they don't. Unbelievable. Unthinkable!"

I lace my fingers together and bring them to my lips, pausing. Robin's fervor is escalating, but I'm feeling more and more calm—almost naturally inclined to apply rational thought, just like Lauren would. "There have to be backups for the patient who's first on the list. A donor heart can't just sit around waiting for a taker . . ."

"There's got to be a way to protect patients from this kind of disappointment. It's wrong! It's insane! How can they do this to you?" She brings her hand to her cheek and shifts her eyes down mournfully. "You've been through so much. I can't fathom why they would . . ."

I raise my open palms into the air. "Okay, okay. I hear ya, Robin. But it is what it is." I've got to stop her right here. I feel shattered by this disappointment, sure, but she is getting upset over a UNOS procedure that I understand and agree with. It is crucial that one or two patients be made alternates or else the donor heart might wind up being wasted, which would be a tragedy not just for one but for many. "I'm not angry," I assure Robin. "I just feel like this missed heart is the knockout punch, you know? I can't hold myself up anymore."

There—I said it out loud: *I can't anymore.*

The sound of it makes my body go limp. As sorrowful as this declaration is, expressing it to Robin brings on a feeling of relief. I've finally summed up in words the exhaustion and pain that have been building these last weeks.

Robin lights up with energy. "All right! So that's why *we're* here! Jill—well, she leaves in the morning—and now me. Let *me* hold you up."

No, no, no—that's not what I need . . .

My reaction is instant and powerful, but I keep quiet. Contained. I remember what Val said about sparing loved ones my quick, sharp reactions. And in this moment, at least, I'm able to heed it.

What do you need, Amy? I demand from myself, silently and without fanfare. *What would hold you up right now?*

I can't think of one thing. I reflect on these past few weeks. Pacemaker firings have taken over not just my nights but also my days—in the form of nauseated exhaustion and heavy-headed haziness. For the first time in all my transplant years, I have started to wonder: Will my mind give out on me too? I've had to make some degree of peace with watching my body deteriorate, deprived of oxygen and kidney function as my heart plunges deeper into failure. But now my brain is on the edge—I can feel it. Line after line has disappeared from my poem repertoire. Casey's social security number escapes me these days. I've had to abandon the remaining episodes of *Scandal* that Joy downloaded for me—no matter how I try and focus, I can't follow the story line from scene to scene anymore. I even had to fill out a form the other day and got stuck on whether my last name is spelled with an *ei* or *ie* (I put down whatever seemed more likely to me at the moment—and realized later that I'd guessed wrong).

I fear that before too long, insomnia combined with the physical pain is going to rob me of the thinking self that has been my steady constant—and I'm desperate to keep this from happening. Survival all these transplant years has depended on my attentiveness to every medical detail. My vigilance has literally saved me from errors and oversights. And now I'm watching myself lose control, my awareness slip away . . .

How can I let anything hold me up? I can't bear an indefinite future in this debilitated state.

Robin herself just bemoaned the endless waiting and uncertainty. She called it inhuman. I agree.

I need to put a limit on it.

I need to know there is a time after which there will be no more fiery black agony burning me alive. And I need to know exactly when this will be. Only then can I keep going.

Yes, this is what would hold me up: a limit on the number of days I must continue on like this.

This idea, I realize, is grounded not just in desperation. I recall at once having read in college about fighter pilots in World War II who experienced psychological breakdowns when observing the daily death toll of fellow airmen. A program was put in place whereby, at the outset, all pilots would be informed of the total number of missions they would be flying. They were assured that after completion they could have a post on the ground indefinitely, if they wished, free from the skies that terrorized them so. The result was an easing of distress and a sharp decrease in the number of pilots deemed mentally unfit to fly. The mission limit gave them something to hold onto.

It seems to me this is exactly what I need as well: a specific end point. Friends can't be part of this. I am going to have to do it myself.

Robin notices my mind drifting and raises her voice a bit. "Look—I know you hate taking the help, but I'm so glad to be here for you. And you know, I . . . I wasn't there last time, and I feel terrible about that."

I hear her concerns, but without focus. I've already begun to muse about how many days—or missions, as I could think of them—I might assign to myself. I muster a quick response, "Robin, it's okay. We were young and—"

But she cuts me off, begging my full attention. "I've asked myself, was I not there for your first transplant because I was stupid and self-absorbed? Or did I just not know how to do it, how to be around a sick person? Our parents taught us how to act at our grandparents' funerals, that's all."

"Well, Val admitted that she had no idea what to do for sick people and their families until she moved to Durham and Sam had that big surgery—'cause all of a sudden people were showing up to do her laundry and fill her refrigerator with groceries and homemade casseroles. Life teaches us. We learn."

"I've learned from you. From your book. I read *Sick Girl* and it crushed me, because I was so absent during that time. And I realized, my gosh, I was such a bad friend! We all were. Why wasn't I there for you?"

It was a forthright, painstakingly candid memoir, *Sick Girl*—I wrote it many years ago about my first transplant and how it felt to live sick and scared when my friends, family, and even doctors expected a simple transplant miracle from me. I didn't describe my friends as sources of support in the book because my relationship with Scott—our courtship, followed by his marriage proposal in the ICU, and then our wedding one year later—was the steadfast center of my universe. If Robin saw herself missing from the pages of my book, she had nothing to feel guilty about.

I assure her that I never for a moment thought she was a bad friend, and besides, "Twenty-five is a long way from fifty."

She wags her finger in the air. "Nah . . . don't let me off the hook. I've felt this for a while—that I need to step up. So when the spreadsheet came out, I said, *I'm not going to make that mistake again!* I was determined to show how much I love you."

"Aw, Robin—I know you love me . . ."

"It's more than that," she snaps, her voice cracking now. "We've reached a part of our lives where we want to own our choices and be proud of ourselves—that's how I see it. We can be better women if we choose to be. And I choose to be here—even if it makes no difference to you. It makes a difference to me. This is so important, oh gosh . . ."

I've never seen her so emotional. Our talks are often characterized by frankness and deep introspection, but Robin's words here seem to be moving toward an unburdening.

She rolls her eyes to the ceiling, gathering her thoughts before continuing. "When we surround ourselves with strong, smart women who have the courage to dig deep into the big questions of life, it's easier to reckon with our own mortality, right? We're fifty. Headed down the other side of the hill. People around us are getting sick—it's not just you anymore, Ame. Some of our parents are dying or dead . . ."

I nod. "Your mom . . ." Robin's mother passed away just a couple of months ago after a long, terrible illness.

"I didn't think I could bear the smell of another hospital after those last months with her. Even stepping through Cedars's doors this morning was . . . Well, put it this way—I wouldn't do this for many people, Ames . . ."

Just then the phone rings. I grab it. "Yes, Emily. Oh, okay. All right.

Thanks for letting me know." By the time I hang up, both Jill and Robin are standing by my bed. "That's the end, guys. The other patient got the heart."

THE MOOD IS just as somber when Dr. Kobashigawa comes in the next morning. Jill has already left for the airport after a tearful good-bye, and Scott is stretched out on her cot now, grabbing a few extra minutes of sleep.

"Morning, morning," Dr. Kobashigawa says, pausing in the doorway longer than usual for his pumps of Purell. He rubs his hands together and then shakes ours. "All right, all right." I don't sit up in bed to greet him. I haven't even changed out of pajamas and into street clothes, or freshened up like I always do before his arrival. "So this heart offer last night, it didn't make its way to you," he acknowledges.

"That was very hard for Amy, Dr. Kobashigawa," Scott says.

The doctor points to the chair next to Robin. "May I?"

She quakes at his asking. "Yes, of course, please, please, sit."

"You know—things work out. They work out, yes, yes, they do," he says, with a new kind of twinkle in his eye. "You see, that heart last night didn't get transplanted after all. No. What happened was—and I'll tell you this without getting too technical—the heart exploded when the surgeon tried to take it out of the donor. It's rare, but it happens."

Robin and Scott gasp in unison. "Exploded? What!"

I stay silent.

"Amy, do you care to explain a little more about it to our novices here?"

Ooh, I could almost give in. He delivers this invitation with an *I know you so well* smile that has eased me through many trying moments in this hospital room, but . . .

"No thanks."

"Well. Let's just say that this heart would not have been good for Amy, or for anyone. So, it's *on to the next!*" He lifts his voice into the slightly raspy, charming range where everything sounds hopeful and so much easier to swallow. *"Heyyy,* you came up number *two* last night—this is *good!* You're going to start getting some heart offers now—*yeahhh.*"

"But they have to match me," I say quietly. "And that's a near impossibility."

"Oh, we've had patients with higher antibodies than you, and they hung in there until—"

"I can't anymore."

Scott comes to sit beside me on the bed and takes my hand. "Amy's feeling like there's no hope. She's been waiting for a while now as a 1A, and it just seems—"

"What happens if I turn off my pacemaker? Those pacemaker guys can come with their magic suitcase and just switch it off, right?" I'm referring to the interventional cardiology team that has stopped by a few times to adjust my pacing settings using a magnet that communicates with a device nestled in an attaché case.

Scott squeezes my hand.

"You need the pacemaker to keep your pulse above eighty. I wouldn't advise turning it off," Dr. Kobashigawa answers.

"Dr. K, the pain came every fifteen minutes last night. *Every fifteen minutes.* And it lasted for about ten . . ."

"It was *brutal,*" Robin adds with emphasis. She was my unfailing support all night, standing right beside me through the hours—extraordinarily focused, tender, and helpful. And now she's stepping up as my witness and advocate, not the least bit cowed by the presence of a doctor who, as far as she can tell, might not be inclined to include an unknown third party in the discussion. She continues, "Amy had to stand by the window most of the night, because every time she lay down, her pulse dropped and the pacemaker fired again."

Dr. Kobashigawa brings his hands together, nods thoughtfully, and sighs. "Yes, I see the increased frequency of episodes on the telemetry report from overnight. Your heart is, ah, barely holding on at this time. You need that pacemaker—though I am sorry for the pain it causes you. I do worry that at some point soon, it might not be enough to keep your pulse in a safe zone."

"I would like to turn it off," I say, calm and certain.

Scott shifts nervously on the bed. "Amy, come on . . ."

I look directly into the doctor's eyes. "I thought about it a lot last night, standing on my giant swollen feet for five hours. I have a right to refuse treatment, and this is what I want."

"What will happen, Dr. Kobashigawa, if Amy shuts off her pacemaker?"

"She will go into cardiogenic shock before too long. Her vital organs will fail. She'll end up in a coma . . ."

Scott bites his lip and turns his head toward the window.

"I'll die," I say.

"*Ho*—not that easy. It will not be a comfortable death," Dr. Kobashigawa advises. He's dropped his chin into his hand, his eyes wide. It's the first time I've seen him worried. "Amy, Amy . . . you have a lot to live for—"

"Please. Don't go into that speech. I've heard it too many times," I say politely, but with resolve. "Believe me, I'm so grateful for all the good I have in my life. I don't want to leave Scott or my son—or my friends or my family. I want to live! You see that I've fought for life these last twenty-five years. But I'm not a masochist. Turning off my pacemaker . . . I see this as an act of love and caring—for *myself*. I think I don't deserve to suffer like this. It's too much pain with too little chance of a good outcome."

"You're 1A now, there will be offers . . ."

"Maybe. Maybe not. But—I've told you this before, Dr. Kobashigawa— I'm not twenty-five years old this time around. I'm fifty. I had time with Scott . . . so much more time than we were supposed to have. I raised my son . . . I was slotted to die when he was in kindergarten. I finished law school. I wrote a book. I got to grow up. I even got to grow a little bit old. It's okay if I have to let it go now—"

"You don't have to let it go."

"I do." I consider telling him about the fighter pilots. But—no.

"Well, it is your choice to refuse treatment. You can have your pace-maker turned off, if that's what you eventually decide."

"I've already decided," I say. He's forgetting that I've had twenty-five years of thought that make this decision an instantaneous one for me.

Dr. Kobashigawa shifts his chin to his other hand and exhales long and woeful. "I need you to do something for me first, please." He grips either side of his chair and leans toward me. "Give it thirty days. I say this because when your 1A Exception was approved, you were granted thirty days at the top of the list. Usually, it's only about two weeks. Now, I don't know why you got the thirty, but I think it's too fortunate to not see it through."

Thirty days . . . *hmmm*. Sounds fishy.

I do a quick calculation in my mind—I remember the date of my 1A approval. It was seventeen days ago. And I learned while serving on the UNOS board that these exceptions are granted for fourteen days and roll into another fourteen if the renewal request is submitted promptly and continues to meet all required medical criteria. It seems to me I wasn't granted thirty days at once; rather, I was granted two consec-utive fourteen-day 1A Exception periods. Nothing notable about that, except for Dr. Kobashigawa's slight exaggeration that rounded twenty-eight days up to thirty.

"*Thirty days*," Dr. Kobashigawa says again, this time with that invit-ing inflection in his voice. "I think it's fate. I really do." He takes my hand in his. "Will you give me the thirty?"

His invoking fate here doesn't convince me. But there is something about this doctor that makes me want to follow wherever he leads—even into fantasyland for a little while. "Okay."

He shakes hands all around and leaves. Scott follows him into the hall.

I open my night table drawer and take out the large pad of drawing paper—the same one I used for the Yeats quote that's set among the array of selfies. I do some quick math in my head—*thirty days, seventeen of them passed already since my 1A Exception was granted.* That makes thirteen days left to fulfill my promise to Dr. K. I grab a red Magic Marker and draw a large circle with a bold number thirteen inside.

I tear off a piece of medical tape, walk to the wall directly across from my bed, and hang my creation for all to see. "The daily countdown," I declare, turning my head to look at Robin squarely.

Her eyes shoot open. "So, you're going to put it right out there, huh?"

"Sure am."

If only Jill were here—I might have set the number inside a big blue triangle instead. She would understand why.

From: Robin Adelson
Subject: Update
Date: April 29, 2014 at 12:28 PM
To: Lauren Steale, Valerie Yablon, Jane Keller, Joy Ceterra, Ann Burrell, Jody Solomon, Leja Babic, Jill Dawson

Hi Everyone,

Amy was very despondent last night and this morning. She was determined not to endure any more nights (or as few as possible). She spent most of the night walking the halls and staring out the window, as this kept her pulse from dropping too low and the pacemaker kicking in with pain. The nights are long and tough and, understandably, she needs a lot of support.

Dr. K came by this morning and tried to lift her spirits. The heart from last night "exploded" and/or "collapsed," as he said. So no one was able to use it. What a cruel feeling though to know a heart was finally available but not good enough. Ugh . . .

This is SO hard on Amy and Scott—can only hope that something good breaks her way really soon.

xo

I'd just twisted my hair into a towel turban and lifted my face to look in the mirror when the first thought hit me: What is being alive anyway? I ignored it and reached for the toothpaste, but then a second thought popped up: What happens when I'm not alive?

Then came a deeper, more disturbing one: What happens when there's no me?

Followed immediately by a fourth that struck me as the creepiest: If there's no me, then I'm not in my head anymore—which means I'll never have another thought!

I put down my toothbrush and shuddered. "Stop, stop, stop," I chanted, and then trilled a few la-la-la-las in a row to unstick my mind. But it didn't work. My head went hollow and I had the scary sense that its contents—that the contents of all of me, really—were nothing— NOTHING!—and had always been nothing, except my thoughts.

I felt I'd discovered a terrible secret about life that I wasn't supposed to know yet: that we're just thoughts in a body—that's all.

So the last and final thought I'll ever have, then, will come right before I die, and after that I'll never think anything ever again. That's what death is.

Stop! Stop! La-la-la-la . . .

I tossed the wet towel from my head, pulled on my foam headphones, and pressed play on my Sony Walkman. A Billy Joel cassette started to roll.

It was 1979. I was sixteen and perfectly healthy.

12 DAYS

My room seems to sink with the sun every day around this time, when the light starts to fade against the always-cobalt California sky. This unchanging weather pattern has made for a drought, Jody tells me. It hasn't rained even once since Scott and I arrived here in late February—or so I've gathered from looking out my window at the same dry sunrise and sunset and all the clear hours in between. Early-morning clouds give way quickly to a dazzling blue that stays straight through to evening, when, sometimes, a wash of pink brushstrokes take over, as has been the case more and more lately. California spring is here, Leja announces daily, along with her recitation of the names of budding flowers and blooming trees she passes while walking the few blocks from our bungalow. I imagine signs of the season's change must be cropping up back home in New York too. The foot-high snow that covered my lawn when I left has no doubt given way to lilac crocuses and yellow daffodils that line the path from my driveway to the front porch. Today is May 1.

It's less than twenty-four hours after Jill and Robin's departure, and three pairs of slippers now rest on top of my bed, each originating from a different point and coming toward the center at angles formed by six denim-covered legs: Lauren's jutting out from the chair by the door, Joy's from the lounger on the opposite side, and mine, a straight shot from the assortment of pillows that prop me up at the head of the bed. There's a new pillow added to the mix today—Mr. Met, an orange-and-blue eighteen-by-eighteen-inch square body with a baseball face sticking out from the top. It was Joy who brought this pillow creature along, of course, stuffing him into her carry-on. "It's a cross-country extension of my Mets shrine," she explained yesterday when presenting it to me.

Lauren might not have understood what Joy meant by this, but I'm plenty in the know about the precise shrine-like arrangement of Mets paraphernalia that has long been her spring routine and obsession. Even though Lauren and Joy are longtime friends, having known each other for over twenty years (Joy shared an apartment with Lauren's then boyfriend, now husband, Lenny, during law school), I doubt they've ever talked about the yearly setup of Mets bobbleheads, buttons, and scorecards in the corner of Joy's DC living room. Joy shares her general high-spirited enthusiasm unrestrainedly, but her kookier stuff gets only a selective reveal. "Let's just say some LA vibes might help our pitching lineup," she added quickly, smoothing over the shrine reference before Lauren had a chance to wonder about it.

I rest my head against Mr. Met and gaze out the same old window. Lauren types rapidly on her iPad, and Joy sits with a stack of work papers on her lap. They've both been hoping I would nap today, encouraging me every hour or so to give it a try, saying "Just close your eyes . . . that's it, off you go . . ." the way a tired mother coaxes her toddler to go down for a nap in the afternoon—because it's good for the kid, yeah, but also because she needs some time to straighten up the house, make some phone calls, and start dinner. I've resisted their collaborative urging, though, and so the second day of this double-friend visit has passed in conversation.

Having covered so much territory already, today's talks have run especially deep and wide, pulling me further and further away from a nap because they felt to me like some of our best so far. At moments, I even allowed myself to disconnect from the subject matter a bit, lie back against my pillow stack, and just take in the feeling of the three of us together—the relaxed exchange and soft laughter interspersed with refrains of *me too* and *that's so interesting* and *I never thought about it that way*. We spoke less about what is concrete and accessible and more about what makes us wonder. By listening openly and carefully to one another's statements of evidence, we affirmed that we all possessed the gift of remarkable intuition. And as we did so, I swear I could smell Val's lavender mist rise up around us.

"You know what Joy and I think . . ." Lauren admitted to me this morning, glancing over at her for permission before continuing, ". . . we've got a feeling—well, it's more than that—we *know* that one of us is going to be here when you get your heart."

Joy chimed in, "Yeah. We are sure that it's going to happen during one of our shifts."

"What a great thought," I said, closing my eyes for a second and imagining what that might be like.

But now, hours later, I'm back to thinking only of the here and now. Hours of conversation have given way to a constructive quiet. With our slippers mingling at the end of my bed, our minds are free to separate and focus individually for the first time today—on one iPad that connects Lauren with her family, one pile of papers that moves Joy through her workload, and one late-afternoon window view that shows me (again) the impotence of hope.

Another day has passed without a donor heart, and soon there will be another night of pain to show for it.

I hate five o'clock.

This is the time of day when my eyes gravitate to a single red light off in the distance; it shows up more clearly in the late afternoon, slowly blinking at me as the sun begins to dip slightly west. At night it becomes a constant beacon that—for a flash of seconds in between pacemaker firings—I allow myself to believe holds promise somehow. I watch and wait for its light to give me a positive sign, but it hasn't yet. And right now I'm thinking maybe it won't, ever.

So much for enchantment . . .

And for that hopeful hummingbird . . .

And my Hebrew name written in the book of life, not death . . .

And Ena's god, who was everywhere . . .

And for the universe that has surely been stormed . . .

It's just a silly light, Amy. It has nothing to say to you. Stop being pathetic.

This snap at myself feels well deserved—for giving in to desperation that imposes believability on nonsense. I make myself a promise: that from this moment on, everything I think and say will be limited strictly to reality.

Except when talking with Casey, that is. I haven't told him about the countdown on my wall, and Scott hasn't either—yet. I imagine, though, that when there are three or four days left, we'll have to pluck him out of the end of his semester and buy him a plane ticket. Meanwhile, Scott and I continue to walk a fine line: trying to keep Casey informed about my medical state without sounding too many alarms that would throw his final college days into a chaotic whirl of grief.

In my mind, I am now facing the most challenging test of our long-held promise to spare Casey the seriousness of my health issues. The minute I took out the red marker to scrawl the first number on the piece of paper, I thought about whether my son should know about it.

No.

It would be selfish beyond all reason.

This countdown is something *I* need.

Casey doesn't need it.

This countdown is the only thing that enables me to hold on.

Casey doesn't need to hear about the fighter pilots.

There is still a chance, after all, that a donor heart might come through. It's a long shot, sure, but to call Casey to my bedside at this point so he can watch Mom count down her life by way of descending numbers posted on the wall—this would be my most punishing last act. I won't do it.

I will spare him.

I will hold on through the missions that remain.

And I will send a final plea out into the universe that somehow, some way, a donor heart will come just in the nick of time and prevent Casey from ever having to know just how numbered these last days were.

I turn my head away from the window and shut my eyes tight. Lauren and Joy are completely focused on the words in their laps.

"I want a DNR," I call out suddenly, startling them.

"What, what?" Joy flinches in her chair.

Lauren's head pops right up. "What did you say, sweetie?"

"A DNR . . . 'Do Not Resuscitate.' I want one of those."

"Not sure what that is exactly," Joy says, meeting my eyes with engaged softness.

"It's a document that tells the hospital not to save me if my heart or breathing stops. I should have done this right away when I got here. But I'm a lot sicker now, and it's looking more and more like it's all going to be over in about ten days anyway." Lauren and Joy raise eyebrows at each other.

"Ah, I think that sign on the wall over there says *twelve* days, missy," Joy quips.

"Okay, *twelve*, har-dee-har. But I'm serious. What are the chances I can get the resident in here to start the paperwork, do you think." This is not a question. I push the nurse call button before my friends can answer—or object.

A voice comes over the loudspeaker above my headboard: "Can I help you?"

"Yeah, hi, it's Amy Silverstein. Would it be possible for the resident to come in for minute? I have a question for him."

"I'll let him know."

"Thanks."

Lauren and Joy sit on the bed beside me now, one on either side. Lauren untucks the throw blanket from around my legs and reaches beneath it to rub my feet. "Let's talk about this DNR," she says. "Why is this so important to you all of a sudden? You're no sicker today than you were yesterday . . ."

Joy opens her mouth and looks up at the ceiling for a few seconds, gathering her words. "And . . . I think Scott should be part of any decision like this, don't you, Lauren?"

"Yes, I most certainly do, Joyous," Lauren agrees, using a nickname from years past to emphasize their alliance. My friends are not speaking with me right now, but rather in front of me—the way parents do when a young child misbehaves. *Tommy needs to understand that he can't throw his broccoli on the floor, right Daddy?* As a mother who has tried this tactic myself, I know that Joy and Lauren's goal is for me to overhear the directive, feel overcome by the strength of two against one, and alter my conduct.

"Guys, guys . . ." I say, waving my arms in front of their faces. "Getting a DNR is not a brand-new idea to me . . . or Scott."

A white-coated body enters the room just then with short, tentative steps, as if on a tightrope. It's Dr. Lunchbox, poor guy—by now, he knows to expect from room 1621 a challenge that is beyond his repertoire of solutions or easy evasions. A smile of relief comes across his face once Lauren turns around to greet him; he is used to her engaging him in calm but highly directed conversation in the hallway. During Lauren's previous visit, I learned to recognize her saying, "I'm going to make a phone call in the hall," to mean, *I'm going to talk with Dr. Lunchbox about this.* Apparently, she has advised the young doctor well. Once or twice, I swear I've heard Lauren's exact words come out of his mouth—and I had to smile at their aptness. I bet he never imagined that a fifty-year-old suburban mother of three would add so much to his medical education and prowess.

"Dr. Baird, I have a request," I say. "I'd like a DNR."

"Oh . . ." His eyes become very round. "All right."

"She hasn't spoken to Scott yet," Lauren offers.

Dr. Lunchbox puffs his chest a little, saying, "There is no require-ment for Scott to sign." His newfound confidence comes from being able to quote established procedure. "Dr. Kobashigawa needs to cosign, actually. It's a form. Pretty straightforward."

"Can Amy change her mind after she signs it?" Joy asks.

"Yes."

Lauren chimes in, "So, if an emergency happened, she could just say, *Forget my DNR . . . go ahead and save me?*"

"Anytime. Yes." The doctor turns his head from Joy to Lauren to me. "All right, then—I'll note in your chart that you are requesting a DNR so Dr. Kobashigawa can take care of it tomorrow morning."

"Great. Thank you."

He steps toward the door as quickly as he can without running, but Lauren jumps up from the bed and follows on his heels, straight into the hallway.

Joy reaches for my hands. "Talk to me."

I give them a squeeze and let go. "I want a DNR, Joy, that's all."

"No, my love. That's *not* all. See, you and I, we like control. And you feel like you don't have control right now, because you *don't*, after all. But is a DNR really what you want here, because I think—"

There is no sign that Joy is going to let me get a word in, so I have to talk over her: "It is what I want, and it's not all about—"

Joy doesn't stop: "—it only gives you something to declare with cer-tainty, even though it isn't right for you—"

I try to break in again, but Joy keeps talking without a second's pause, so I speak right along with her: "But, Joy, it is right for me . . . I had a DNR at Columbia—"

She keeps on. "—so, really, you should wait on this, think about it for a few days," she says, "and talk with Scott about whether he thinks—"

"*Joy!*" I shout, finally. "You're wrong on this one!"

I've known Joy to power through with unstoppable determination when making a point—going on and on without heeding any contributive words, even ones that agree with her. And I've learned to sit back and let her speak it all out; it's what she's used to doing at her job, after all, where critical business outcomes rely on her exceptionally informed opinion. But survival is my critical business, and I'm the one with the expertise that comes from hard work and a long, long tenure.

"Joy . . ." I say again, with less intensity, "if I don't do the DNR now, it leaves open the possibility that I'll have to call out for one in an emergency situation. And if that happens, no one will take me seriously—there will be stress and chaos and they'll say I'm not *of sound mind*, or whatever the requirement is."

She lowers her eyes. "Yeah, okay, that makes sense . . ."

"But you're right about one thing . . . this is about control. I have to act now so I can have control later. I don't want them coming at me with machines and defibrillator paddles. And now's the time to protect myself from that."

Joy pauses for a few seconds. "I hear you, I hear you. I do. Really. But"—she springs from the bed and claps her hands together once—"you know what I think it's time for? Focusing your mind on life outside of this room!"

Oh boy. Here's that exaggerated Joy again—the one who spun through my kitchen a few months ago in a flurry of determination to make tea. Joy can be the best listener and partner in figuring out the most complex challenges—but pushed to the emotional brink, she can bulldoze through a conversation and whip her can-do spirit into a frenzy. She wiggles her fingers at me now, moving them toward my forehead and then away, feigning power to plant a message in my head.

"I think you've been cooped up too long, and you're forgetting that there's sunshine out there and people smiling and enjoying the day—just like you're going to do after your transplant."

Oh—and now for the encouraging *after your transplant* pep talk. Joy knows better than that; she must be feeling terribly desperate.

Her intensified state, then, can't just be about the DNR. Joy must also be reacting to the number on the wall that greeted her with its stark gravity when she arrived yesterday. And this is why she ran so long and tenacious on her no-DNR speech: she means to rearrange reality for me—proclaim that I'm down in the dumps because, after spending so many weeks here in the hospital, I can't see the sunshine future that awaits me when I finally get out.

But, of course, I do see the future—and this, precisely, is the problem.

"When and if I get out of here, I'll just be going back to a sick life, Joy. The same transplant body I had before. And this is a *re*transplant, so it's going to be even more complicated."

"How do you know?"

"How do I know? Seriously?" We've talked so many times about the antibodies and cancer risk that threaten second heart transplants like mine. "Oh, come on, Joy . . ."

"Well, I say come on . . . *out of this room*! And into the California sunshine! Never mind the future—this is what you need now!" She's really on an optimistic, overwrought roll. "We've got to find you a way out of here. We will talk with Dr. K . . ."

This won't help. I've already spoken with him about it several times, and he agreed with Dr. Lunchbox: I would need accompaniment by a doctor and nurse, which isn't feasible given the crucial need for full staff at all times on this heart failure floor. Scott, however, came up with an alternative last week—a secret scheme whereby he and my friends would take matters into their own hands (no doctor or nurse needed).

"Never mind Dr. K," I tell Joy. "You should talk with Scott. He's got a plan to actually sneak me out of here. It's totally not allowed, of course, and so I don't think I should do it. Rules—"

"—are made to be broken!" Joy says. "If there were ever a time to break 'em, it's now—I'm just saying . . ." She gestures toward a small plaque that Robin brought and set on my night table:

Well-behaved women rarely make history.

—ELEANOR ROOSEVELT

"Maybe. We'll see," I say.

"No, no. This is exciting! I'll talk with Scott about it tonight—can't wait!"

"Can't wait for what?" Lauren is back. She's been in the hallway for a while—must have given Dr. Lunchbox quite a talking-to for accommodating my DNR wishes so swiftly. That's the look on her face, anyway—peeved—like the mother who wanted to stop little Tommy from throwing broccoli but couldn't, and then her husband went ahead and gave him the ice cream he'd been clamoring for.

We all want things our way—Lauren, Joy, and I. With our kids, our jobs, ourselves. Sometimes, even with each other.

We're all after control.

11 DAYS

Justin comes in with a double Valium dose for me tonight—five milligrams. Up to now, I've taken a mere two and a half milligrams (and even this dose only a handful of times because I am still struggling with drugging away my awareness). But sleep deprivation has been pummeling me harder than ever lately, suggesting definitively that my heart has now moved beyond the pulse-sustaining abilities of my pacemaker. Night after night, I am able to get about two hours of sleep, and not all at once—and the same goes for whichever friend or friends are by my side. Last night was the worst so far; Joy and Lauren took turns standing with me at the window, and even this didn't prevent my heart rate from dropping. So this morning, Scott, Lauren, and Joy had a powwow with Dr. Lunchbox in the hallway, and this led to a visit from a palliative care doctor and a quick prescription for an increased dose of Valium at bedtime.

"Okay, I've got a big five m-g's for you tonight, Amy," Justin trumpets. "You want it now or should I come back later?" He stands to the left of my bed, clicking away at the hospital computer. I turn my head and watch the prominent muscles of his forearms fire as he enters notes about the brief physical examination he's just given me. Every time there's a shift change, the nurse assigned to my room checks my lungs (*breathe in and out . . . and again . . . good!*), my ankles (a few presses against the bloat yields a rating from one to four), and my heart-beat (*uh-huh, okay . . .*)—this part of the exam always transforms Justin into a man of uncharacteristically few words.

"Five milligrams will be no different from two-point-five," I say. "The first pacemaker firing will wake me up, and that will be the end of that. I'm not going to take the Valium, Justin."

Lauren and Joy pipe in at once—

Nuh-uh, you're takin' the Valium, girl . . .

We talked about this . . .

You need your sleep . . .

"Justin, dear, can you please tell our stubborn friend that Valium is happening tonight," Joy says.

"Yeah, Justin. Let's gang up on her a little," Lauren adds.

He's still at the keyboard. "Ladies, ladies . . ."

"You're interrupting Justin's nightly report . . ." I say.

Sorry, Justin!

Oops, didn't mean to . . .

He logs out of the computer, and the Cedars-Sinai main screen appears. "Now, Amy," he says, "you want my opinion?"

"Yes, we do, Justin!" Joy demands. "Please do share your great wisdom with us."

"Yes, abso . . . lutely!" Lauren trills. "Let's all have a nice long talk about the virtues of Valium . . ." She pats the seat of the empty chair beside her. "Can you sit with us for a few minutes?" Justin, as a favorite night nurse, has already spent multiple late-night hours chatting in my room during Joy and Lauren's previous visits. With Cedars's highly manageable nurse-patient ratio on the sixth floor, Justin is usually assigned only one or two other patients at the most, and typically they're elderly and sleep through the night. Once he's finished giving them their medications, there's often time to hang out with us.

He glances at his watch. "Yeah, I think I can sit. Thanks for the invitation." He smiles wide with those great white teeth. "It's an honor . . . I feel like I've been tapped to attend the *it* party . . ."

"Oh, we're *it*, all right," Joy boasts. "I mean, who's more fun and interesting than us three?"

"Well, there's a guy down the hall who's got a rash on his butt . . ."

"Ooh, do tell!" Joy kids.

"Well, it's not a rash, exactly. More like boils . . . round red things filled with pus and—"

"Ew!" Lauren squeals.

"Gross, Justin, ugh," I say.

He breaks out a devilish grin, "Just kidding! I don't have a patient like that. So I guess I have to agree with you, Joy, yes. This room is the most fun—and all of you are the most fun, of course."

"Ho . . . wait a second," I warn. "You might have to leave me out of that designation. I haven't been the most fun today. I made an arrangement with the palliative care doctor this afternoon that has turned out to be, shall we say, very *unpopular* with my friends."

"Oh, so you met with Dr. Moore from palliative?"

"Yeah."

"Seems like a decent guy," Justin says. "He's new here . . ."

"A newbie?" Joy rolls her eyes, "Oh jeez. Well, Amy sure broke him in quick. Gave the guy a real shocker today, I think."

Justin's cell phone rings—it's the Cedars-issued phone designated for intrahospital calls from patients and doctors during his on-duty hours. He answers right away, "This is Justin. Yes, yes. Okay, I'll be right there." It's a patient down the hall. Justin has got to run. "But I'll be back . . ." he says, striding toward the door. "I've still got your five milligrams, Amy . . ."

"Hear that, Ames? He's still got your Valium, ready to swallow," Joy says. "But, you know, I'm actually glad you didn't take it yet . . . so we can be sure to get Justin back to sit with us some more!"

"Did you notice he's got new glasses on tonight?" Lauren says.

Joy snaps her fingers. "Yeah, handsome. Too bad he's getting engaged, darn it."

"What's the latest on that?" Lauren asks.

"Ames, has he mentioned it lately?"

"Uh . . . eh . . . what's that?" I haven't been paying attention. My mind is stuck on the comment Joy made about the palliative care doctor—that I *gave the guy a real shocker.*

When Dr. Moore (or Andrew, as he insisted I call him) came to see me, he must have known he would be meeting a patient who was in great pain and probably quite near death—because that's typical of palliative care clientele. I have to believe that Andrew's training and years of experience readied him for an encounter with challenging patients like me; his is not a specialization for physicians with vulnerable sensibilities who cave at a curse word or anguished wail. Palliative care is meant to ease patients' worst suffering.

And besides, Joy and Lauren went out for coffee when Andrew stopped in, leaving Scott and me alone to talk with him until the tail end of the conversation, when they returned.

"Why do you think Andrew was shocked?" I ask Joy now, skirting her question about Justin's engagement.

"Oh—okay, well . . ." She switches gladly to this new subject. "When Lauren and I walked in, he seemed uncomfortable. He was twitchy . . ."

"Like you made him really, really nervous," Lauren adds. "And did you notice—his tie was kind of shaking."

I laugh. "Yeah, it was, actually." Andrew's skinny tie lay so flat against his ultra-slim-cut fitted dress shirt, it seemed to move with his heartbeat. He was trim and neat, soft-spoken, and prone to overexpressiveness of his eyes—but all of this, I noticed, was the case from the get-go, even before our discussion took off like a shot in a most unpleasant direction.

"He was helpful," I had explained to Joy and Lauren earlier, giving an overview of the conversation they'd missed. "We landed on two important decisions . . ." Scott sat back in his chair and laced his fingers together in front of his lips, allowing me to explain.

"One—I absolutely need sleep." I'd told Andrew that the nighttime pacing had worn me down to a level of exhaustion I've never experienced before. The longing to close my eyes and rest without cardiac agony was so intense that I'd begun to wonder what delirium might feel like and whether I might be approaching it. "So he gave me a prescription for double the Valium dose, which will start tonight," I told them.

It was music to Lauren and Joy's ears—*That's great . . . love it . . . super idea . . . Justin will be thrilled . . .*

"And two—just before I turn off my pacemaker, palliative care can come in and give me enough sedating medicine so I won't have to feel myself slipping into that awful cardiogenic shock Dr. Kobashigawa keeps mentioning."

No response.

"It's essentially pain management, that's all," Scott assured them.

"And who knows, maybe my heart will pump on for a few days without the pacemaker—and a donor heart might come through just in the nick of time."

"What if a donor heart *doesn't* come through?" Lauren asked.

Joy nodded in agreement, frowning. "Yeah."

"Look, guys, that decision has already been made." I pointed to the sign on the wall where I'd written the number eleven in Magic Marker first thing this morning. "The only thing that's new here is the addition of pain relief and sedation." Lauren and Joy squinted skeptically. "The palliative care team is not turning off my pacemaker. That's *my* doing. They're just responsible for keeping me comfortable . . ."

Scott sighed loudly and pushed himself up from the chair. "I think I'll go back and do some work for a few hours." He gathered the newspaper and his briefcase, kissed my forehead, and walked toward the door with his eyes on the ground. "See you all later, okay?" Lauren and Joy stood up to hug him. Taking their seats again, they assumed an unusually rigid posture: elbows tight to the body, hands clasped, lips pursed and set. My friends were frozen by what they'd just heard. The way their intense gazes shifted searchingly, one to the other and back again, made clear to me what a rare and panicked moment this was for them. What I was seeing take effect for the first time in these two commanding, capable women was the inconceivable shock of inefficacy.

Andrew might have stammered and jittered a bit, sure, but this seemed to be characteristic for him, not a reaction to the situation. He handled my emotions and wishes with grace and skill, determining how various pain relief modes might help me and then explaining my options with cool neutrality. It was Lauren and Joy, though, who were shocked—not so much by the requests I expressed to Andrew (they'd heard them many times before), but rather by the palliative care response to them.

"I have to say, this whole scenario, how it's all going to work . . . it . . . it just . . . surprises me," Lauren admitted, pressing her lips together.

"Doesn't Dr. K have to sign off on it?" Joy wanted to know. "Isn't this a cardiac matter?"

The ease of the process spooked them. For my friends to hear me say *no more* and at the same time recognize that I can actually achieve this end through calm, rational, and alarmingly feasible means was unprecedented. Scarier still: there seemed to be nothing they could do about it.

Lauren and Joy had better footing when trying to put up barriers in the past—though I didn't always recognize their actions as such. When I was in the throes of deciding whether to have the double mastectomy or to let breast cancer take its course, courageous Lauren engaged me in a conversation about how I thought I might die. "You're not going to sit around and let cancer ravage your body—that would be awful for you," was her first shot at dissuading me at the time. And when I agreed with her that, no, I wouldn't choose a long painful death, she pushed even further: "Let's talk about ways you might end your life, then."

All right . . .

"Pills?" I proposed, halfheartedly.

"Not a good idea. You might only make yourself super sick, and then start vomiting. Someone would find you and you'd wind up in a psych hospital."

"Well, shooting myself or cutting my wrists is out—I could never do that . . ."

"Agreed . . ."

We went through a few more options, with Lauren keeping her emotions in perfect check and playing the role of helpful friend who can hear anything without getting the slightest bit rattled. And by the end of our talk, it seemed clear to me there was no good way to lay down my life at the foot of breast cancer. It was the same point Dorothy Parker had made in a poem I memorized in college, where she describes her own disposing of impractical death routes (drugs, nooses, rivers, razors), concluding that *you might as well live.*

I had the mastectomy. But, like Dorothy, I suppose, choosing to forgo death felt more like a shrug than a determined mission. This shrug was a surgery that saved my life, of course, and it was Lauren who had the guts to risk talking me through death options in order to reach this end. But her support felt genuine to me, and our talk was so extraordinarily brave (even the very best of friends aren't apt to venture into such territory) that Lauren didn't seem like a barrier maker that day; she was more a magnificent pair of ears—perhaps the most open ears that had ever heard me.

Joy had also done her share of listening with remarkable composure and daring. When she flew to visit me in New York back in February, she encouraged digging right into the *New York Times* article about the New Mexico man with the sick heart who sought the right to end his life. The similarity between his case and mine did not intimidate Joy or dissuade her from putting on her lawyer's hat—and asking me to do the same—in order to think through all the details of how I might follow in his footsteps. Bringing our minds together in a serious way to make sense of such a far-fetched possibility made me feel that Joy and I were on the same side of things.

But now I'm not sure. The shock that Lauren and Joy perceived in the palliative care doctor during our conversation is a reflection of their own surprise and discomfort, I think. For all the bold and exceedingly open talk we've had about death over the last few months, I now realize that beneath it there has always been an assumption of safety. My friends know that my goal has never been suicide, per se. It is, simply, a longing for the right to stop fighting like hell—at some point. So this means that guns, pills, and even "death with dignity" were never going to fit the bill; my aim was omission, not commission. Lauren and Joy understood this deep down—that there was a safety latch in place—and so, perhaps, their apparent bravery was easier in the face of these unlikely scenarios. But now, as I've landed upon a more tangible, rational plan, their boldness falters. The pacemaker-turnoff scenario has flipped the latch.

There was no hiding my friends' desperation to walk things back. "How about we bring the palliative care doctor in here first thing tomorrow and we all talk with him together?" Lauren suggested just after Scott shuffled sadly out of the room.

"I know *I've* got a few questions for him," Joy chimed in.

"And I haven't had a chance to write him into my book," Lauren added lightly, holding up the notebook where she'd kept a diligent record of all occurrences and observations.

"It's hard to get a hold of the guy," I said. "He might not come back around until after you're both gone."

Lauren's eyes narrowed. "Huh—well, you know . . . maybe that's even better. Gives you time to think about things. Right, Joy?"

"Mmm-hmm, I agree with you, Lauren. Time is good. Time brings clarity . . ."

"I already have clarity," I said.

Joy pursed her lips.

Lauren shrugged. "I guess *we* don't," she said softly.

They wanted to be the very best friends to me that they could—this was for sure. But they also wanted control.

Now that I've reached my limit, my stop-fighting-like-hell point, and put in place a clear and doable plan for comfortable sedation, the question arises: Do Lauren and Joy dare support me?

JUSTIN RETURNS AS promised, dropping immediately into the chair that he sprang from half an hour ago. "Okay, so where were we?" He places his Cedars cell phone beside him.

"Amy was just about to take that double-dose Valium . . ." Joy says.

"Was I?"

"Yes," Lauren agrees. "Justin, can you try to talk some sense into her?"

He slaps both his hands against his chest simultaneously and smiles. "Me? I'm not sure I'd want to try to talk Amy into anything."

"Thank you, Justin. I take that as a compliment."

"But what do you say . . . I hang out here for another, oh, I don't know, twenty minutes—and then I give you the Valium and you go to sleep?"

"Sounds like you're trying to barter," I say.

"*Ahem, ahem* . . . As Amy's lawyer, I'll counter your offer and add one stipulation," Joy says. "Make it thirty minutes—*and* you agree to fill us in on the latest details of your engagement."

"Deal," he says.

I pipe up while they shake on it, "Hey, I didn't agree to—"

Justin bats his eyes at me, cajoling his way past my objection. "So you already saw a picture of the ring, right?" Lauren tells him she hasn't, so he retrieves his personal cell phone from his pants pocket and brings up a photo. "I picked up the ring two days ago. And my plan is to propose this weekend."

A communal squeal erupts: *Justin! So exciting!*

"Tell us, tell us!"

"First thing, I've got a dinner reservation at Melisse in Santa Moni—"

"Wonderful!" Joy bubbles, interrupting him. "Good choice. French. Perfect!"

"And I thought I'd propose beforehand because—"

"Beforehand, of course, do it beforehand!" (Joy again.)

"Because . . . she will want to call her parents and her sister, and that would mean making calls all through our dinner. So, I got a hotel room on the beach—"

"Romantic!" Joy hunches forward, landing her forearms on her knees. "And are you going to pop the question *there*?"

"Well, I was thinking it might be best if . . ."

A wave of weariness rolls over me.

Suddenly, I couldn't care less.

I'm too weak and tired to stay focused. My attention weaves in and out of Justin's proposal plan—he's saying something about setting the ring box on the couch and letting her discover it, which sends Lauren and Joy into a chorus of objections . . .

You lost me there, Jus . . .

Yeah, you've got to be more inventive . . .

This is how you should do it—so you call the hotel in advance, and . . .

Joy sets out her vision—I hear the words *room service* and *silver serving tray, chocolate-dipped strawberries* and *champagne*. Justin diffuses Joy's insistence with a series of polite *okay, okays*. Lauren asks whether he plans on kneeling, sitting, or standing when he asks for his girlfriend's hand.

Justin drops abruptly from his chair and tries out his future proposal pose with flourish. "Well, there's our answer," Lauren says, "and I like it!"

"Me too!" Joy chimes in. "And how 'bout you, Ames? Are you with us on the new ring-on-the-tray plan for Justin's engagement?"

I force my eyes fully open. "Wha? Yeah, yeah, sure. Sorry, everyone, I'm exhausted. But don't let me stop the good time—feel free to keep chatting."

Still with his knee on the ground, Justin pulls a blister-packed pill from his pocket and thrusts it toward me: "May I propose . . . five milligrams of Valium?"

Laughter all around—then stillness. Justin's arm remains extended. "Okay, okay—I'll take it . . ." I say. Lauren pops up at once and retrieves a bottle of water from the minifridge while Justin empties the pill into a little white cup, seizing the opportunity. "I like Joy's idea about the room service and the silver tray . . ." he says, handing me the cup while prattling on. I take the pill with a sip of water, and swallow. "But I will tell you this"—he takes the now empty cup from my hand—"there can't be chocolate-dipped strawberries, because that's what I did the first time I was married—"

"*What, what, what!*" Joy shrieks, raising her hands to the ceiling and jumping from her seat. "*You were married before?*"

"Well, yeah. It was a short and unfortunate—"

"And you're just telling us this now!" Lauren howls.

"Oh, Justin, *Justin!*" Joy cries, "You're going to have to tell us everything—*right . . . now!* But wait, wait . . . ha-ha-ha . . ." Joy collapses onto my bed with laughter. "Amy just swallowed five milligrams of Valium! You know how fast that stuff works on her—she'll be snoozing before you get to the first juicy detail. For the love of God!" She yanks my torso forward and starts pounding my back with her open palm. "Spit up that pill! Spit it up! "

Even I'm guffawing now.

"All right, Justin, you're just going to have to spill the beans fast," Lauren demands. "So what about this first marriage of yours?"

Justin complies. "It was about ten years ago, while I was working on Wall Street in the finance industry . . ."

"*You worked on Wall Street!* That's bonkers! Amy, who is this imposter posing as our Justin? And we thought we knew this man!" Joy nudges my arm repeatedly, but I feel myself drifting off already, slowed by the first syrupy seeping of Valium heaviness—and it makes me sad. I know there's no real chance for sleep tonight, even with this double dose.

One hour and I'll be up with pacemaker pain. What stupid hope they all have . . . and how silly I was to give in. Damn it, I've lost control . . .

Even through the sedative haze, I latch onto an idea and begin to brood. Something about this situation rings familiar—and suspicious. All this talking and listening and laughing tonight, all the unusual lengths gone to by a nurse who's willing to spend an hour in my room sharing details of his upcoming engagement: it led to me taking the Valium I hadn't wanted to take. And this harks back to times in the past when Lauren and Joy devoted themselves to me with greatest effort, delving into the most intrepid discussions about how I might rise to the challenge of my body's ills—or not. But rather than supporting me in moving toward the particular goal I had in mind, my dear friends (and now also, it seems, Justin) actually succeeded in moving me toward the particular goal *they* had in mind instead.

Support is not always pure, as I see it revealed now. Support may be kind and generous and well-meaning, but it navigates with a compass of its own and, sometimes, a deliberate hand on my rudder.

From: Lauren Steale
Subject: Hi and love
Date: May 2, 2014 at 6:40 PM
To: Joy Ceterra

Joy, I want to tell you that your presence here with me was something to behold. You made Amy feel loved and cared for and heard and important and visible. And you are one Florence Nightingale. Really, I will say that I believe I am pretty good and attentive and way up there, but you my friend are enviable and I am in awe of your patience and way.

Being able to spend time with you the past few days was just so nice. Of course the circumstances were not ideal but they certainly did provide an opportunity for us to be together and really talk, and I cherish our sister time. It is something we will always remember—and I am grateful for Amy and her large circle of special friends.

I love you Joyous and so appreciate our friendship.

Xoxo

10 DAYS

Come on, we're going, and that's that . . ." Scott insists. I've been resisting his pleas to sneak out and grab a few minutes outside, and now he's taking charge. "It'll be good for you. Today's the day." He retrieves my sneakers and kneels down to help me put them on.

"Scotty, I don't feel right about it," I say while he ties and double-knots the left one.

He turns his head to speak over his shoulder to Ann, who sits on a chair behind him. "Amy is a big-time rule follower from way back."

"Ah, I get it," she says. "Not like the rest of us."

"It's not just the rules—I'm not sure I can walk all the way to the elevator. I haven't been able to get past the Swan-Ganz lately." I'm referring to the colorful poster in the hallway that shows the mechanism of the Swan-Ganz catheter—it's only about ten feet from my door. "And then once I step out into the lobby, how far is the exit?" I've never seen the layout of Cedars's lobby, not even when I was first admitted to the hospital since I was taken straight from the ER to my room on a stretcher. "What's it like down there?"

"There's a lovely little courtyard just outside the door. It's not far . . ."

Scott doesn't seem to be taking into account that five steps—*just five!*—make me lose my breath; that's why I've refused his offers to walk in the hallway lately.

"How many steps, do you think?"

He finishes tying the other sneaker and reaches for my hands to pull me to standing. "I don't know . . . twenty, thirty maybe? You can do it. I'll be right there, holding you the whole time . . ."

He doesn't get it—holding me won't make a difference. I'm not afraid my legs will give out; it's my heart that won't last the forty steps. I need a wheelchair, not a firm arm around my waist. But okay, this sneak-out is going to happen whether I'm comfortable with it or not. "This is going to be so good for you," he repeats, walking backwards and leading me toward the nurse call button.

"Wait . . . I have to take off my telemetry leads." I reach under my shirt and feel around for the stick-ons where the EKG wires snap in. "One!" I call out, peeling the first one from my chest and handing it to Scott. "Two . . ."

"Hey, Scotty, while you're doing that, can we go over my role here just one more time?" Ann calls out from the chair at the far side of the room. "I want to make absolutely sure I've got it down pat."

"Of course. First thing—Amy's going to press the nurse call button and tell them she's going to take a shower, so they'll alert the telemetry folks that she'll be off-monitor for a little while."

Ann pays careful attention. "Yes, right, got it . . ."

"I'll turn the shower on before we walk out, and close the bathroom door," Scott continues, "and you'll go ahead of us into the hallway, making sure the coast is clear. When you see that we've got a safe path to the elevator, you wave us on . . ."

"Okay. I check for nurses. Signal when to go. I will do that. Yes."

"And then I'll run Amy to the elevator—"

"Run?" I say.

"I'll get you there, honey. Don't worry."

"Now. Tell me again what I should do if someone comes in while you're out," Ann asks. "I will do *exactly* what you say . . . and, uh, I promise I won't snooze on the job this time . . ." She raises her giant Starbucks cup and smiles sheepishly. "I'm gonna be sipping one Venti after another today, you can be sure of that . . ."

Ann means to make up for what happened last night: she slept through every one of my pacemaker firings, and this has left her feeling not only regretful but also baffled. As a very light sleeper, Ann assured me that she would be up in a flash whenever I needed her. But when the first scorch of pain ripped across my chest at midnight, I snapped awake and glanced in Ann's direction, and made a quick decision not to call out to her. Seeing her curled up on the cot in peaceful sleep, it dawned on me that I had woken too many exhausted friends over the past few weeks, and that I should try to rely on myself for once. Ann did not in fact fail me last night by sleeping soundly through the night; rather, she inspired in me a new awareness.

Even so, Ann remains convinced that the mishap was her doing. She is well aware of the protocols outlined in the emails and how her first night in my hospital room diverged from them. As I see it, though, a bit of nonconformity during my sister-in-law's visit is both fitting and welcome. In contrast to my tightly wound and routine-focused friends and me, Ann is refreshingly spontaneous and intuitive. She goes with the flow and the feel of the moment with an easy confidence that I admire and sometimes try to emulate (with only modest success).

It is because of Ann's unique influence that I have dared to hold the reins of control more loosely at times and to take an unexpected path every now and then. She's the only friend of mine who still possesses a few hippie sensibilities alongside her more conservative ones, moving seamlessly between the far-out and the predictable. A modern dancer by profession in her early life and a therapist in her current line of work, Ann operates on the soul level by seeking substance over form. She tends toward platform clogs (comfortable), the do-it-yourself hair dye (less ado), and the calm, balanced mothering of her two *Free to Be*

You and Me daughters (more harmonious). There is a glow of joy in her home that is enviable—an absence of pressure that invites long, serene exhalations. I've been fortunate to settle into the rocking chair in Ann's living room often, where I feel myself floating above it all.

Married for the past twenty years to Scott's brother Gary, Ann has been a constant and vital presence in my life. By her seamless, worry-free approach to slipups—which she usually laughs off easily and waves away with a swish-flip of her hand—my dear sister-in-law, who is older than I by a few years, reminds me of my much younger self, when not every action had monumental consequences and not every inaction felt like such a great big deal. In her take on life, a missed opportunity only opens the chance for another try at it. I've reflected on this quality in Ann a lot lately, contemplating whether I might cut myself some slack—maybe even bend a rule or two. What harm could come and who would know?

Last night in my hospital room, however, Ann set out to do a very specific job that had been perfected and set out in detail by her predecessors. She brought full intention to it and relied on her night owl nature to help see things through, but she knew the minute she woke this morning that all had not gone according to plan: "Uh-oh . . ."

"No, Ann, it's okay—really."

"*I didn't*, did I?"

"Yeah, you did. But it's fine. I figured it's about time I try to get through the pacing on my own a bit. There's nothing anyone can really do to make the pain go away faster, so—"

"Just can't believe I slept through—"

"Ann, all the girls would have slept through if I didn't scream to wake them. But last night, I chose to try to handle it myself."

She nods thoughtfully. "Okay . . . I understand."

"And I did okay, see that? Good to know that I'm not a completely dependent mess. . . ."

It strikes me how much I want to put Ann at ease. Things have changed—*I* have changed—since Jill occupied the cot as my first friend visitor over a month ago. At that time, it was all about what I needed from those around me—most specifically, getting them to understand. But since then, the understanding has come to flow both ways. Where I used to be so hungry to take in empathy, now I am just as eager to give it.

I put my hand on Ann's shoulder and look into her eyes. "Do you know how happy I am that you're here?"

She swats at me, half smiling. "Yeah, yeah. But I promise you—I will stay up the entire night tonight so you won't be tempted to let me sleep . . ." She pauses, smoothes her hair back nervously and sighs, as if doubting her own pledge

Only reparative action would soothe her. So when Scott came in this morning ready to put his sneak-out plan into action, Ann rose to the occasion at once, hell-bent on carrying it out perfectly.

She listens now to Scott's reiteration of her role with unblinking eyes.

"The shower will be running and the bathroom door will be closed, right? So, if a doctor or nurse comes in, just tell them Amy's still in the shower and they should come back in about twenty minutes."

"Right. I got it."

"Thanks, Ann," I say, signaling for Scott to pull the two telemetry leads off my back. "I still feel funny about this plan, though . . ."

"What's the worst that can happen? You get caught and we don't get to do it again."

"Again? I say we do this *once* . . . That's all I have the nerve for."

"You got this, Ames. You got this," Ann assures me.

"Okay, press away . . ." Scott says, handing me the nurse call button.

"Hello, can I help you, Amy?"

"Yes, hi. I'm going to take a shower. My friend is here with me, so I don't need any help. I'm taking off my telemetry now, okay?"

"Thanks for letting us know. Enjoy your shower!"

"Thanks."

"All right, here we go," Scott says. "Ann, you head out first and tell us if it's safe to come." He walks me to the door, and I secure a yellow surgical mask over my mouth and nose. Ann steps into the hallway and he peeks out after her, watching as she walks to the intersection where we will turn toward the elevator. "That's a thumbs-up—*let's go!*"

"Holy crap," I murmur as he clasps my hand tight, leading me out the door.

We reach the sharp left that leads to the elevator. Ann is there, again with a thumb pointing up. She runs ahead of us and pushes the down button in the vestibule—a move that was not articulated as part of Scott's plan but is terrifically helpful. By the time we arrive, the elevator is already there and waiting for us. "Pressing the button—great idea, Ann. Great!" I say, stepping inside swiftly.

"Good luck, you guys," she says, and the doors close.

We're not alone in here, Scott and I. There are a few others heading down with us in the elevator—two nurses, a doctor, and two people in street clothes. I've got a mask on, but this is not necessarily suspicious since transplant and chemotherapy outpatients wear masks in hospital settings. So do visitors who might have a cough. What I'm afraid may give me away, though, is the way my mask keeps flapping smack up against my mouth when I breathe in—fast, fast, fast. I'm gasping. Scott notices, and grips the length of my arm from elbow to wrist. He pops his eyes at me—*I got you, I got you . . .*

We step out into the lobby.

People moving, everywhere! There's a Starbucks kiosk—*Look how long the line is!* Everything is fast and bustling and incredibly alive. I hear the street sounds from close up now. And there's light . . . I'm moving toward natural light!

I take off the germ mask as Scott pushes open the door. We step outside. "And here's the courtyard," he says, "just like I told you. See the outdoor sculpture? This one's a fountain, but they turned off the water because of the drought. We can sit. You want to sit?"

I don't respond.

"Amy, you all right?"

I nod. I'm still struggling for breath. But this is not what catches my words in my throat. I am overwhelmed. All of this life around me! All this air! And open space! And the sunshine, oh, *the sunshine* . . .

"Is the sun this bright in New York?" I ask Scott. "I don't remember sun like this. Oh, honey! I forgot how beautiful . . ." I'm crying.

Scott takes me by the arm and leads me to a ledge where I can sit. I close my eyes and tilt my face to the sky. "Ahhhh . . . *so good* . . ."

"I told you so. This is just what you need."

"You were right, Scotty. I feel like I'm dreaming . . ."

"We can't stay long, though," he says, taking my hand with tenderness.

"Okay, okay. But I know it's *here*. And now I know I can come see it. Feel it on my skin. I've been in a hospital room for so long . . ."

"Give me a kiss," he says, tapping my chin with his finger.

I open my eyes and then close them again, and we kiss.

I feel the strange sensation of a real smile stretching my mouth, my face.

Happiness.

This is all it takes—five minutes under a bright, clear sky and one kiss from Scott, and I am supremely, utterly, immediately blissful.

Scott turns to me again. "This is what you're doing it for—for us . . . for our life together . . . for little moments of sunshine and blue. That's all we need to be happy. You're going to get that heart, Amy. We have to keep hoping . . ."

"Yeah, okay . . . okay," I say, blinking away tears as he guides me up from the ledge and toward the hospital lobby doors.

"You can do this again tomorrow," he says, smiling.

"I want to . . . I really do . . ."

"Then we will."

I secure my germ mask in place, and we step inside the building, leaving all color and light behind us. The lobby is dim and the ceiling feels awfully low. We step into the elevator and Scott presses six. It's the first time I've seen my floor button pressed. I realize with a start: this is what Lauren has done . . . and Jill and Joy and Leja and Robin and

Val . . . and Jody and Jack and Ann . . . and my father and the rabbi. And Scott—my wondrous, adoring love and lifeline—who has pushed that button more than anyone, all day long, every day, for so many weeks. How strange to be standing here with him when he presses it yet again, delivering me back to my waiting list sickbed.

But maybe over the next ten days, I hope, a surgeon carrying a cooler with a donor heart packed in ice will press this same button, lift up through this same elevator shaft, and save my life.

Oh, to be able to live. To stand in the sun again with my Scott.

From: Joy Ceterra
Subject: Hello Friend
Date: May 3, 2014 at 9:28 PM
To: Amy Silverstein

Hi Amy . . .

I have to say, you have such wonderful friends. I'm sorry it has taken these past few months for me to get to know them on a deeper level. They are so warm and lovely and supportive even to me these past months—part of me wishes I had stayed in NY and had the opportunity to get to know you all as a group even better. It makes me happy to know you've been surrounded by so much love in your life—Scotty of course, but these wonderful people too. Each so different, but all wound together in their amazing love for you.

Today . . . I know you felt the sun—*the sun* . . . something I take for granted. For me, sun is medicine for my soul—so it made me happy to know you were able to feel its wonderful energy today. But I can understand that that feeling it must also have made you feel cheated— that something so simple in concept as the sun on your body is such a rare treat for you as you wait and wait and wait . . . I wish you could feel the sunshine every day to remind you of this simple beauty that awaits you if this heart were to come.

I'm glad you've had time with your wonderful Annie. I imagine she's been a comforting soul, helping you feel cared for and loved.

I'll see you Wednesday afternoon. I look forward to our talks. Tonight—
please try for just a little more sleep with the Valium. Be kind to yourself,
friend.

With love,

Joy

AFTER AN INTENSELY caffeinated day, Ann feels prepared for the night
ahead. She sits in the chair beside my bed and vows again to stay up-
right and awake all night long. Nothing I say can dissuade her. "I've
only got one more night here to do it right," she tells me. "I'm not going
to risk falling asleep again. After last night, I don't trust myself."

"It's *me* you shouldn't trust—I decided not to wake you."

"Did you decide not to wake any of the other girls?"

I pause, but not for long—I can be honest with Ann. "All right. I
didn't have the heart to wake you, no pun intended. Can we please drop
it now?"

She shrugs. "Okay. But you should feel free to shut your eyes and go
to sleep. Don't let me keep you up just 'cause I'm sitting straight like a
scarecrow here." She has settled herself into a chair beside my bed with
an iPad on her lap.

I turn on my side and face her. "My pacemaker is going to keep me
up. Give it fifteen minutes—watch. That's why I dread going to sleep.
It's the worst part of my day. So I'm in no rush to close my eyes."

"Want to talk, then? We can chat if you want . . ."

"Yeah."

"Okay, good."

"But let's not talk about waiting for a donor heart, all right?"

She chuckles. "Fine with me."

"Let me tell you, then, about your sweet daughter Abby. Do you
know—she's texted me every night . . . *every single night* . . . to say 'I love
you' and good night? And she sends the goofiest pictures. Got one the

other day of her on the toilet, in a bathroom stall at school. 'Thinking of you, Ames,' she wrote, or something like that. I laughed out loud."

"She's a nut muffin." Ann smiles. "And oh, she loves her Auntie Amy. Maddy too. Both my girls adore you."

"I adore them."

"You know, Ames, I'm going to need your help with Abby's college applications in the fall. I want to talk with you about some schools that might work well for her—where she can play soccer *and* get academic help if she needs it." Abby has a learning disability and has to work hard at writing and organization.

"She can do it," I say. "I have full confidence in her smarts." I witnessed Abby's natural aptitude and study capacities just a few months earlier when she was required to memorize a hefty chunk of *Romeo and Juliet* for English class. Ann delivered her to my house for a dose of Auntie Amy's literary memorization technique. I taught Abby my method, and she caught on immediately and with enthusiasm, so we went ahead and memorized all the pages in one sitting. I called Ann and told her she could come pick Abby up early, happy to report that she had the material down perfectly. She's a memorizing whiz, actually. "And if a kid can memorize, she can do well in any subject. Period," I said.

Abby earned the best grade in the class on recitation day. Still, Ann was no less concerned with finding just the right college where Abby would be sure to thrive—and then there was the matter of prodding her to complete her college applications on time and with full effort. And now this challenge was close at hand: Abby would be finishing her junior year in just two months, and already there had been college-counseling seminars at her school, as well as assignments in English class that were prompts to prepare for the standard college application essay. "I'll be handing her over to you to help with some editing in the fall, of course," Ann tells me now.

If I'm here for it, I can't help but think.

"Actually, she told me she wants to write her essay about you,

Ames . . . about the texts she writes you every night and how much she admires you. She's so proud of those texts, you know."

"She should be. You know, when you're young, you want to run away from people who are scary sick, right? Don't you remember being little and passing a cemetery and holding your breath? What Abby is doing is pretty remarkable—reaching out to me every single night. I tell you, it's so much more mature than the way my twenty-five-year-old friends acted when I had my first transplant . . . some of them headed for the hills and we never spoke again. Abby is brave."

"She loves you."

"Yes, but she's got something in her, that girl. She's—*uh-oh* . . ."

Heaviness.

A pulling in my chest.

And here it comes . . . the searing pain from shoulder to shoulder.

"Ann—I'm pacing, damn it. Ow, ow . . . Oh my God, *ow* . . ."

She jumps to her feet. "Should I, uh . . . what can I do for you? I, uh . . ."

"This is worse than ever," I gasp. "Holy crap . . . *ouch* . . . *ouch* . . ." I shift my legs over the side of the bed and push myself to standing, hoping it will make my pulse rise. "Help me, Ann. I'm too weak . . ."

She slips her hand around my waist, and I lean my body weight against her. "I got you."

"*Ow* . . . *ow* . . . it's ripping through my chest!"

"Should I call the nurse?"

"Uh . . . no . . . well, maybe yes . . . I don't know. The pacing has been a lot worse lately. Let's, uh . . . give it another couple of minutes . . ."

"Can you stand it?"

"I have to stand it, Ann. This is what my life is now . . ." I press my lips together and feel my eyes well with tears. "But just for ten more days now. And then, no more. No more."

Ann blinks long and shakes her head. "Just hold on, hold on to me . . ."

"Oh, Annie!" I cry, collapsing against her shoulder. I begin to weep.

"Sorry you have to do this . . ." Up until this moment, I've tried hard not to let myself cry during nighttime pacemaker firings because it seemed only to make it so much harder on everyone. Friends have attended to these episodes with a loving but mostly logical, problem-solving approach—each woman with her own method and goal of getting me through, it seemed, and an air of confidence, whether real or skillfully feigned. Ann, though, is not capable of methodology; she has no guile. She is simply present, with wide green eyes, not even attempting to mask the tortured twisting of her facial expression or the lack of self-assuredness upon seeing me so ill. Had Ann come earlier in the spreadsheet calendar, I would have been an easier sight to bear and challenge to rise to. But timing and fate have placed her at the closest point to my end and the furthest point from hope; she is here to catch my near-ultimate fall—and I am so comforted by her presence. Her body movements channel serenity—a dancer's grace in the way she elongates her neck and folds toward me ever so slowly with a gaze of acceptance. I am reminded of a yoga teacher's whispery instruction to imagine floating on a lotus flower—*There's no need to change anything . . . You're just as you need to be in this moment . . .*

"I just love you so much, Ann," I say, gripping her tighter.

"I love you too, Ames."

After a few minutes, the pain subsides. She leads me back to my bed and pulls the blanket up to my chin. "There you go." She pulls her chair up close beside me, takes my hand, and holds it for a long, long time—ten minutes, fifteen, twenty. We sit wordlessly, staring with unfocused eyes. I turn my head toward the red blinking light without imaginings tonight; the only good luck beaming toward me is my choice to end this waiting list ordeal.

Out of the silence comes an admission. "I feel selfish," Ann says, splaying out her arm toward the wall of photo faces. "You say sorry to me . . . sorry that I have to be here with you. But you know what? I am so glad to be here—it's a gift to me to be able to help even a little tiny bit. Because you've given me so much . . . and the girls too.

Helping them with things I'm not too great at—the memorization, the writing . . ."

I assure her that it has been my absolute pleasure. Over the years, I have jumped in (often without Ann asking) to help her daughters work toward certain aims—whether a timetable and checklist for college application deadlines, preparation for the Regents Exam in biology, or Shakespeare memorization. My nieces are always appreciative and on-task, acceding to my instructions and study techniques much more readily than my own son. Plus, they're girls—what fun that is! I give them the short skirts I no longer wear and the cosmetic samples that come with my wrinkle cream purchases. There has been a particular joy in contributing to their lives and watching them blossom over the years. "And Ann, you could have done all of it without me. You *will* do it without me, if that's the way it turns out . . ."

"It can't turn out that way, okay? You're not replaceable. The way my girls respond to you . . . and admire you. You're such an amazing addition, a wonderful . . ." She begins to sob, ". . . part of—*sniff*—my mothering. You round me out as a mother. Yes, that's what you do, Amy." She wipes away tears with both hands.

"Ann—" I turn toward her and open my mouth to say something lovely in return, but my thoughts freeze up. In truth, it is Ann who has rounded me out as mother—showing me by example how I might ease up on expectations of Casey and support his seeking of a broad variety of paths in life rather than imposing the narrow, predictable ones that are familiar to me. But what is first and foremost in my mind at this moment is the most essential way in which she completed my experience as a mother: by inviting me to attend the births of both of her daughters.

"Since you'll never be able to give birth, I thought maybe you'd come to mine so you can experience it," she told me, eight months into her pregnancy with her first child.

It was, to me, an unimaginably sensitive, kindhearted, and selfless offer to invite me into the privacy and intensity of her first birth. Along with her husband, Gary, and a midwife, I would be the only other attendee, she said, and I accepted with the deepest appreciation and awe. A few weeks later, I drove from New York City to a suburban hospital where Ann, Gary, and the midwife were already hard at work in what would be a very long (and very loud) birthing process that had me immediately aghast at my opting in to this fantastic, horrific spectacle.

Ann was screaming—I mean *screaming*. The incredible decibel level of it reached me the minute I stepped off the elevator, and it intensified to such a piercing howl as I approached the door to Ann's room that I couldn't bring myself to open it. Willing strength through the moment, I stepped inside and witnessed the next several hours of my dear epidural-refusing sister-in-law waiting for her damn cervix to expand, yelling and grunting and, at moments, weeping. The louder and more raucous she got, the quieter and more excruciatingly slow and deliberate the midwife became—and oh, how I wanted to smack that Mother Nature birthing ambassador in her stoic little face! "Aaannn, yoo-hoo, Aaannn," she cooed, responding to Ann's shout of *"I'm going to break in half!"* Then the midwife spied me crying in the corner. "Hey, you," she said, losing her übergentle-soul facade for a few seconds. "Stop with the tears."

I did. But I couldn't bring myself to do much else to help matters. Since I had no experience in dealing with other people in severe pain, let alone the agony of natural childbirth, all I could think to do was stand aside and let the drug-free delivery technique takes its good, sweet time. Gary's attempts to soothe Ann were met mostly with wails and curse words—another reason, I thought, to steer clear. It wasn't until the midwife called me to her side and dropped one of Ann's heels into my hand to hold up in the air (just at the moment the baby's head was crowning) that I found my place in that arduous scene: it was to observe birth, just as Ann had wanted for me. Ann put me there not to help her, but simply to have a thrilling experience of womanhood and motherhood that I otherwise would not.

I watched baby Madeleine come into the world with a final push and howl—and then silence. A cut of an umbilical cord. A newborn placed on her mother's chest. A smiling Ann and tearful Gary.

Joy. Pure joy.

The absolute miracle of birth.

But what struck me most that night, and what I carried with me when I floated out of the door that I'd entered in trepidation hours earlier, was this: the incomparable power and strength of women. Watching Ann bring this baby through her and out of her and then *letting her go*—the first excruciating release in what would be a series of letting-gos over Maddy's lifetime—seemed to me the most astounding, painful, magnificent feat I had ever witnessed. To see all that Ann went through so that this baby, this child, this human life could breathe on her own and have a life of her own—oh, the sheer mightiness of it. My sister-in-law was a warrior woman. She was brave and daring and persevering. She was, in the most powerfully visceral way, a mother.

And they say heart transplant is miraculous. I say the bringing forth of life beats it by a mile. And I only know this because Ann allowed me a front-row seat—twice.

"You've made me whole as well . . . you know, having me there when the girls were born," I tell Ann now, allowing honesty to carry my thoughts aloud instead of trying to find just the right words.

"I was lettin' it all hang out. What a sight!"

"I don't remember any of that. They say you forget the worst of it, right?"

We laugh just a little.

Ann lifts her gaze back to the wall of selfies and sighs. "Ten days, huh? Do you really have to? I mean . . ." She frowns and sighs again. "I support you, Ames, but I'm sorry, I can't . . . I don't know how to leave here tomorrow knowing that I'm probably never going to see you again."

I shrug. "Maybe I'll get lucky?" I say halfheartedly.

"But, but . . . Abby . . . she's writing that essay about *you* . . ."

And Scott's going to have to summon Casey here in a couple of days.

I cover my ears. "Ann, please don't."

8 DAYS

ere comes Jane.

Smiling so bright.

And I want to say sorry to her immediately because I know I'm not up for whatever she's got to offer. The spreadsheet keeps sending dear friends my way, but I can't say I am actually receiving them anymore. With Ann's departure this morning, I feel I've lost all animation and motivation, and it shows.

Where I had been rising up eagerly for long, meaningful exchanges and reminiscences with friends in my hospital room, now I'm fine with silences and small talk. I don't seize the opportunity to find humor anymore—the Dr. Lunchbox name has lost its mischievous gleam for me. Strolls in the hallway have shortened to just a few steps outside my door and back again. And when I manage somehow to slow-step some twenty feet outside my room to the giant scissor (the art poster that used to spur laughter because of its likeness to an upright penis), all it stirs in me is anxiety at how much more out of breath I am now than when I first stood in front of this image, laughing.

Being in my company is without a single bright spot, and this is why I worry about Jane's arrival. As perhaps my most exuberant friend, with a can-do nature that rivals my own, Jane would be likely to seek out my spark and expect to light it—because she's done so in the past, and handily. She's got that rousing way about her that catches you up like a charm and makes you feel like you're the reason for that special gleam in her smile, whether you're a close friend or just a casual acquaintance. Watch Jane walk down the main shopping street in our town, and you might mistake her for a popular mayor; a one-minute stroll from the drugstore to the butcher shop turns into a fifteen-minute saunter for Jane because she will be stopped by no less than a dozen people along the way—*Jane! Jane! Hi!* I've walked down the street with her many times, so I know. Jane greets and is greeted by more people in five minutes of errand running than I am in two years of the same. Someone comes over to chat with her on our path, and I observe a lesson in affability, trying to put my finger on just what's at the core of it. In the almost thirty years I've known Jane, I still can't name it exactly. But whatever it is, I totally get the power of it—and the power has surely gotten me.

On many occasions, Jane has shown up to my medical smackdowns just in time to flick the switch that rebounds my spirit, getting me up and out for coffee, praising me for charging through yet another challenge with guts and smarts. Jane sees the best and the strongest in me, and heaps on the accolades in such a direct, assured way that I find myself agreeing with her: *You're right Jane—damn it, I really am optimistic and resilient!*

But, see, I'm not anymore.

All Jane has built me up to be is likely to come tumbling down during this visit. And I worry her sparkle will have no effect.

And yet, look at this—Jane has actually got me walking in the hallway now, far from my room, which I'd rather not be. But it's her second day here, and suggestion has turned to insistence. "Let's go, okay, okay? You can do it, right?" she asked a few minutes ago, opening the closet to find my sneakers before I could confirm my willingness to walk. I felt the automatic rallying response trigger within me, as Jane must have hoped. But what's different this time is that my body may not be able to accommodate my will—or hers. Last night was awful. Nearly constant pacing kept us up and anguished. Justin was off duty. There was nothing but pain and longing for sleep on both our parts, while Jane kept stalwart vigil.

I know this walk is beyond me. I've barely been able to make it ten steps from my door lately, and now, with Jane holding my arm, I find myself halfway around the square expanse of the sixth floor. Jane doesn't seem to mind at all when I stop again and again to catch my breath; she talks animatedly through each panting pause, bringing me up to date on her kids and on the latest goings-on back home in our town. "They say Whole Foods is coming in. Supposedly, they signed a lease for the space near the high school," she says, ushering me right along, even though the girls' emails have detailed how weak my heart has become. Jane knows, and yet she moves assuredly—unhindered, undaunted—across the white tile floor because she has determined that it's the right thing to do. Jane believes getting out of my room is good for my body and mind and will show me something that I need to believe right now, i.e., that I can still walk like I did when I first arrived here.

I'm not sure she's right on this one, though. I look at Jane now— she's got her face lifted, turning left, then right, as if checking out new shops on Main Street. She breezes along with poise and grace. An image comes to mind—it is perhaps one of the strongest memories I have of Jane, one that has left an unforgettable impression on me. We're walking through an airport, my family and hers. We've just taken a ski trip. Scott and Casey move along fine, as do Jane's husband and son. And then there's Jane's four-year-old daughter, who erupts into a tantrum and refuses to walk until Jane gives her something (what it was, I don't know, but man, did that girl have a pair of pipes). The rest of us stand in place, watching and waiting for this parent-child standoff to resolve so we can continue on as a group. Jane renders a final, powerful no, causing her daughter to collapse to the ground and grab hold of her mom's right ankle. "Okay, let's go!" Jane calls out, and onward she marches, dragging her wailing daughter along the trodden terminal floor.

Oh, how much easier it would have been just to let the kid have her way, right? That's what I would have done—I, who stuffed a quick Popsicle into toddler Casey's hand in the park years earlier, just so other mothers wouldn't judge my railing three-year-old. But Jane held firm—she was not going to cave to a tantrum, not even in the airport. She made a quick determination of what was right and acted fully in line with it, because the best outcome for her daughter (and, perhaps, herself) was not to heed this kind of behavior. And Jane carried it out seamlessly; not only did she walk with aplomb while lugging forty pounds of a kicking and screaming child who had hold of her ankle, she also did so with head held high, looking ahead for a kiosk where we could buy water bottles and magazines.

Jane is the calm, resolute mother, sticking to her plan of action with awe-inspiring confidence and competence. And she is doing the same here with me today, I realize, as the exceptionally self-assured friend who carries out with determination what she deems best under trying circumstances: getting me the hell out of my room.

I have to stop for breath again. "Whole Foods! You're—*gasp*—kidding me?" I finally answer, once I've got enough air. "Really? I'm going to—*gasp*—die, and now they put in a Whole Foods?" I say this in fun, but the disappointment beneath it is real; all the years I've lived in the suburbs, I've haven't had a good place to buy fresh fruits and vegetables. I'm actually annoyed at the thought that my ill-timed demise will mean missing out on this new development. "Of all the luck," I add, kidding just a little bit.

"Oh, stop it. You'll be pushing your shopping cart through the aisles like the rest of us."

If Jane had said this to me even two weeks ago, I would have jumped on it and forcefully impressed upon her how the odds are stacked against me. Up to now, I've been quick to shoot down optimism from any visiting friend who dared toss it cheerfully in my direction. But there's no point in keeping this up anymore. My ending is all but assured. And while I wondered plenty in March and April, when friend after friend flew home, whether it was the last time I would see them, now in early May this thought has become a certainty: I will never see Jane again.

Sorrow stings in my throat as Scott's words rise up in me again. They ask a question that begs to be answered this minute—not in a general way, but with regard to the friend with whom I stroll right now and for the last time: *How do I want Jane to remember me?*

With my arm linked through hers and feeling the struggle in each step forward, it occurs to me that maybe by insisting on this challenging walk, Jane is actually helping me project an image that will remain after I am gone. It's as if she is determined to flick on my light switch and illuminate the attributes she has long admired in me: resilience, audacity, guts . . .

But if I appear to glow here in this hallway with the best in me on display one last time, it's because of Jane. Not me.

"You're unbelievable," she said to me earlier this morning, and so many times in the past, and yet she has the utmost belief. I don't want her to find out that, truly, you can't believe what you see about me.

I pull back my shoulders, trying not to drag so much on her arm for support.

"Hey there, you! On a morning stroll—I like it, I like it!" a nurse calls out, waving as he comes toward us with steps so quick that I feel a rush of air as he passes. A doctor in a sleek suit and tie stands at a hallway computer and looks up at the sound of the nurse's voice. His eyes fall on Jane and rest there with a twinkle for a few seconds. I'm not surprised.

"Did ya catch that doctor checking you out?" I ask her once we're far enough down the hallway to be out of his earshot.

She pulls me closer to her and laughs.

"I'm serious. The guy we just passed. In the beige suit. He took a long, good look at you, boy—"

She waves me off. "Get out . . . maybe he was looking at you!"

"In my yellow germ mask? I don't think so, Janie. Even without the mask, no one's lookin' . . . I'm death walking."

"There you go again. Stop it, would you? You happen to look pretty darn fabulous—considering. Yeah, you're a little tired around the eyes, but I gotta say, you don't look anything like I've read in those nightly emails—which I chose to take with a grain of salt, by the way. I appreciate the girls' sending them, but I'm my own person, you know, and I'll evaluate the situation myself when I set my eyes on it, thanks very much."

Jane is, for sure, a straight shooter. I like this about her. "Grab that door!" I call out. "Let's go in *there*!" A nurse has just stepped out of a key-only entryway, and Jane catches it adeptly now before it closes. "Check this out. I've only been in here a couple of times, mostly with Leja when I first got to Cedars and was able to walk this far."

"You walked just fine," Jane says. "You're doing great." I ignore that comment and focus instead on the exceptional surroundings. Jane and I find ourselves standing alone in the middle of a glass overpass that connects two Cedars buildings. The view on either side is wide-open—the Hollywood Hills stand out in the distance against blue sky while, closer in, tall palm trees line San Vicente Boulevard as far as I can see toward Melrose. I can even make out the nearby corner where our bungalow sits: a white dot nestled within tall walls of greenery. The feeling of this hallway is exquisite spaciousness, quite unlike the more contained sense I got when I stood in the courtyard with Scott a couple of days ago. Looking far and wide now, I can almost imagine being able to breathe in all that air—there is so very much of it between ground and sky. "I want to be out there," I say, not realizing I've spoken this thought aloud.

"You will be."

"It's not looking that way, Jane."

"Far as I can tell, you're not going anywhere. I know what the doctors say and what the waiting list challenges are, but I'm sorry . . . I just don't think it's your time. Look at you! You're full of vitality, Ames."

So I can't die because of how I look?

My breast doctor, whom I met at Starbucks just a few months back in order to get her to call off the cops, said something remarkably similar to me. When our discussion hit its critical point that day, just minutes into our peppermint teas, my doctor articulated the reason she thought most salient and vital for not letting breast cancer be the end of me: "Amy . . . you just have too much vitality to die."

"*Oh?*"

"You know, I see patients with no hair, looking so ill and wasted away. But you—for all you've been through—you're still so very, very full of life! You look too good to die."

That was her best argument?

As Val would say, *Good grief!*

What should it matter how I look on the outside?

Here was this renowned breast surgeon sitting across the table sans white coat in a crowded Starbucks and unwittingly showing me the downside of my insistence on always looking my best whenever I go to the doctor. It had long been my self-imposed rule that sickbed pajamas and matted hair must always give way to jeans, a flattering sweater, and some well-placed makeup. Lights, camera, action: it's doctor time! Decades of medical experience have taught me that doctors tend to have a greater affinity for patients who look like they've got a good shot at a favorable outcome. It is a double-edged sword, though, because the more life a doctor sees in you, the less he or she can imagine you without breath and heartbeat. Even doctors with a wealth of knowledge in their brains and years of experience on their side tend to be more swayed by what they see with their eyes.

Appearances are, I've come to understand, that powerful.

I tell Jane I need to start heading back to the room. "But thanks for pushing me to get all the way here today. Great to feel my legs moving again. And I forgot how much I love the view."

"See that? It's great. Maybe you'll do it again when Joy comes."

"Maybe," I say, trying to sound breezy about it. But right now, I'm feeling a distinct pulsing in my neck—I imagine it's the vein that Dr. Kobashigawa has been using as a teaching tool to demonstrate my "restrictive allograft physiology" (as he calls it, enthusiastically). I've glimpsed the very apparent, bulging purple protrusion every time I brush my teeth in front of the mirror, but I've never once actually sensed its thumping. Overly aware of it now, I feel instantly dizzy and hot, but I force a smile; I don't want to disappoint Jane by stopping in my tracks and whimpering for a wheelchair.

Perhaps picking up on my sudden preoccupation, Jane cozies up to me with that sense of can-do support, and so I push on—small steps, frequent stops. I spot a few white-coated gazes gravitate in our direction as we make the trek back; my sparkly friend Jane is a sight for sore hospital eyes. She also achieved an incredible feat with me today—the sixth-floor hallway loop.

If I can make it back to my room.

Jane's cell phone rings. She retrieves it from her back pocket. "Oh, look, it's Rob . . ." (her husband). "Hi, honey, I'm just here taking a nice walk in the hall with Amy. Yeah—she's a walkin' machine, doing pretty darn fabulous, considering . . ." She gives my arm a squeeze of encouragement. Seconds later, she wraps up the call and tells me, "Rob sends his love . . . and he said he just wrote you an email . . ."

"Oh, okay . . ." I'm concentrating—*right foot, left . . . right foot, left . . .* Just then, we pass an empty stretcher parked in front of the nurses' station, and my thoughts shift—*I gotta lie down, I gotta lie down . . .*

But just a few steps more and, look at that, we've reached the door to my room. I pull off my yellow mask. Jane walks to the chair and falls into it with a contented thump. Within seconds, I'm settled in bed and feeling safe again amid the Hawaiian leis, the streamers, the tie-dye. My body tingles with the strangely pleasing aftereffect of exercise. The pulsing in my neck vein quiets. I look over at Jane, who's smiling as she taps the keypad of her iPhone.

I exhale. Slide my feet under the fleece throw blanket. And in the peace of this moment, it dawns on me—*How lucky I am . . .*

The harrowing hallway loop looks different from here—more like a small victory, or even a big one. A final hurrah orchestrated by my amazing friend Jane. She helped me do my best. Gave me something to be proud of.

From: Rob Keller
Subject: A few things
Date: May 5, 2014 at 2:54 PM
To: Amy Silverstein

Dear Amy:

I know Jane is with you now, and while I fully expect to see you again, I didn't want to risk not telling you directly a few things. (Does email count as "direct"? I guess it'll have to, for now.)

You have lived a great life. It is in many ways heroic and historic. But while your disease has occupied so much of your time and energy, I don't think of you as defined by it. I think of you as Amy, period: your sense of humor and irony; your creativity; your quick and distinct laugh; your generosity and friendship; your truth telling, even when it isn't convenient.

You've touched many people in ways you'll never know. You've forced us to examine our lives and ask, *What would we do if we were Amy?* And I don't mean if we faced your health issues; I mean, in our own lives, with our unique challenges: Why can't we be more courageous? Why aren't we more demanding and more direct? Why aren't we more loving or more giving, in the face of struggle and pain?

I don't know why. But I think about it a lot and I assure you, so do your family and friends.

You've lived a life that matters, one of great consequence. You've made people take notice. We are profoundly the better for it.

But when I think of you, my enduring thought is that you've clawed your way to a thousand ordinary moments with Scott and Casey, and your friends. Much of them, far as I can tell, with an abundance of love and happiness. That's the stuff of an extraordinary life—the ordinary is what's extraordinary. It's what any of us would want.

It's those countless moments that stitched our friendship and our lives together, Amy, and it's why I love you.

I will see you soon.

Rob

Jody comes in a little while later. Scott and I drafted her to help with a sneak-out today, and we've got an eleven o'clock rendezvous plan. He is going to meet us downstairs in fifteen minutes; it's Jody's job to deliver me there. Jane is today's trusty lookout.

I talk my trainees through the procedure that Scott and I put in place when Ann was here. We go over each step with grins on our faces. "This is fabulous," Jane says.

"I was pretty scared the first time, but now I figure, what can happen to me?" *There are only eight days left on my wall,* I want to add, but I don't. I'm conscious of the unfortunate fact that Jane, whom I respect and love a great deal, landed a spot far into the spreadsheet order and so has come at a late point in the game, where I am focused on nothing but turning off my pacemaker. I have to try hard not to bombard her with it.

I give the countdown to action. "Okay, girls, three . . . two . . . one!"

Jane dashes down the hall and gives us the all clear. Jody and I follow—onto the elevator we go, down to the lobby, and out to the courtyard.

Bliss.

I sit on the ledge, close my eyes, and put my face up to the warm sun. "Jody," I croon, "this is heaven on earth."

"I'm so glad, Ames." I hear the scuff of her sandals against cement ground; Jody is pacing, nervous. It is one thing to sit alone in my hospital room with me when no other friend is there and Scott is caught up in a business call back at the bungalow (as Jody has done nearly every day since I was admitted to Cedars in March), but to be my lone company out here on the plaza, breaking hospital rules, leaving my heart unattended by a telemetry monitor—this feels like an enormous responsibility. And a dangerous one.

"Scott will be here in just a couple of minutes," I say, bringing my head back to level, opening my eyes, and glimpsing her very troubled brow.

"Yeah, yeah. It's all good," she says, and I appreciate that she's faking it. Because, for me, this is truly *all good*.

I lift my face to the sun again. "This is so fantastic. I could die right here and now, and it would be fine with me."

"Well, it wouldn't be fine with *me*—I'll tell you that," Jody shoots back immediately with all seriousness but, at the same time, tinged with that comedic edge that infuses most of what she says.

I laugh a bit.

"I'm not kiddin' ya', Ames."

"I hear you, I hear you . . ."

Just then, I see Scott emerge through the lobby doors. He bounds toward me cheerfully. "I love to see you out here! It fills my heart . . ." He kisses me on the cheek and then reaches out to hug Jody. "Thanks so much, Jo."

"I'd like to say it was my pleasure, but this, Scotty . . . this racks my nerves a little, I have to tell you. And then your wife, she says she could die right now and that it would be okay with her . . . I mean, I'm havin' a real ball out here . . ." She's joking again, and Scott and I get a good chuckle out of it. Our friendship with Jody—and with Jack too, who has been here almost every day as well—has come so far since we first arrived in California. Thrust into the highest-pressure circumstances of life and death, we've glimpsed one another in the extreme: the fury of my silence after the pacemaker procedure; the rare display of Scott's last-straw loss of patience with me; Jody's disintegration into fretful, wide-eyed pacing; Jack's unabashed tears as he lay beside me one afternoon, realizing that our hallway strolls were no more. How could the clash of horrible ordeal and intense hope not speed us past the usual steps of relationship progression? With our deepest emotions laid bare, we couldn't help but relate in a way that eludes even the closest of friends.

The strength of our new bond makes me feel happy and sad at the same time: I have come to love Jody and Jack just in time to start missing them.

"You want to head home now, Jo?" Scott asks.

"I do."

"All right, then. I'll take it from here. Hope to see you soon."

"Yeah, I'll be here in the morning."

"Joy's coming tomorrow," I say.

"Great! I'll email her tonight and see if she wants me to pick her up at the airport. Can't wait to see her."

Joy and Jody . . .

New friends.

Good friends, now.

Transformed by fate, it seems. There's no escaping it. All the women who've spent long hours in this room have been sorted and realigned, awoken and opened up, challenged and embraced by this tragic and beautiful coming together. Our friends have expanded, and we are expanded as friends.

But to what end? Will the whole of us be undone when the countdown hits zero?

I stayed in the bathroom long enough for Jane to call out to me, "Everything all right in there?" and I told her I'm fine, just giving my face a good scrub.

"Today is exfoliation day," I said, as if I actually knew what day of the week it was.

I wasn't scrubbing. I was thinking.

Sitting on the shower bench and contemplating the day passing without a donor heart and the night of relentless pacemaker firing to come.

I didn't want Jane to see my despair.

She piped up outside the bathroom door, "Well, I love the Bliss Fabulous Foaming Face Wash . . . It's mild so I can use every day, but it's also got a great . . ."

I stood up, walked to the mirror above the sink, and leaned toward it.

Man, I look like shit—dry, wrinkled, drawn, beaten down . . .

I sighed.

Then, in a flash, I lifted my forehead, eyebrows, cheekbones, and the full expanse of both my lips, and I forced a big, bright smile: this was me doing my I'm well face, as I'd named it long ago. I had amused myself many times with this trick over the years, catching my reflection in the mirror at random moments and seeing illness in such obvious display, and then erasing all traces of it—poof—by elevating every inch of my face at once, forcing a healthy smile upon a stricken droop.

Remarkable. I was still able to do it even now, just about one week before my dying day . . .

My dying day—for fuck's sake.

I'm going to turn off my pacemaker in seven days.

And then what?

I pushed my face right up against mirror and gave myself an intense once-over—

Who am I?

What happens when there's no me?

Giving palliative care a nod for sedation will be my last act . . . my last thought.

Stop . . . stop . . . stop!

La-la-la-la . . .

I shut my eyes tight and called out to Jane, "I use the Bliss face wash too! It's the best."

6 DAYS

There comes a time in the course of a fatal illness when the desperate routine that has worked to suspend it just above the depths doesn't work anymore.

There is little comfort now in having Joy in a chair by my bed all night long.

She has stopped taking notes on my nightly pacing jolts because there are so many of them now that they've become an incalculable stream. And each one lasts for what seems like twenty or thirty minutes straight, until my heart eventually begins to budge toward a safer pulse rate. Pain episodes have become constants, as has the need for soothing. But no friend can scratch a back that long, and even if she could (Joy surely tried last night), incessant tactile motion dulls my skin's sensitivity until the sweep of fingers across my back feels like nothing at all.

So we try standing by the window. But by three a.m. we're too sleep-deprived to talk, our mouths and ears shut down, and we become swaying posts with fluttering eyes. The Hawaiian leis and skirt grass rustle beneath Val's slightly open window, tempting Joy and me to launch a few frustrated swats and hurl a curse word at them. And even just the thought of that blinking red light out in the distance there makes me want to throw up.

Too little sleep and too little hope rattle the foundations of this room now. Every thing and every soul—every act and word and presence of mind brought to it by nine women who've held on and on in the name of resolve and a newfound understanding of love and friendship—are shaken now. Exhausted. Perhaps even beaten.

A number is set inside a circle on the wall.

And in the glaring despair of its message day after day, my friends' positivity has begun to fade. It occurs to me that perhaps they've even begun to grieve me. A pang of sadness clutches my stomach now as I realize: the loss of my friends' hope feels like my loss as well. But there is nothing to be done about it.

I look out the window along with Joy and find one of those rare blue-pink-orange watercolor sunsets we've come to love—but neither one of us bothers to mention it. "I'm sorry," I say.

Joy turns to me slowly. "What, hon?"

"I said I'm sorry, but . . . I want you to know that you shouldn't have any doubt about whether I am going to turn off my pacemaker in six days. Really. Please take me seriously."

"Amy—I do . . ." She draws in a deep breath, holds it, and then exhales long and somber. "I hear you. I believe you. I see what's going on with your body, how much worse your heart has become. I see the level of pain." She pauses, lifting her eyes to the ceiling to ward off tears. "You have my support."

"Thank you." I pull two tissues from the box and offer her one.

Just then, Leja lets out a squeak of anguish. She crosses her legs and hunches forward, burying her face in her open hands. I sit up and reach toward her, but Joy intercedes, touching my shoulder and recapturing my gaze.

"Tell me, Ames . . ." she continues, tenderly, scooting her chair right up against the side of my bed. "Is there something I can do for you?

Something to prepare for what's to come? Do you want me to write down what you'd like done after you're gone? Maybe you want to give your journals to someone. How about the book you were working on last year—save or destroy? You want me to get some stationery so you can write letters to Scott and Casey?"

"I've written them already. Scott's got them, actually. But yes, it would be great if you could make a list of a few things. Thanks."

Joy reaches into her tote bag and pulls out a yellow lined pad. She climbs on the bed and sits alongside me, sharing my pillows. "Okay, shoot . . ."

"Well, I think I'd like to give Jill the necklace I'm wearing . . . and, um . . . I would like someone to destroy my journals, actually, since they're pretty private . . ."

"You sure? Maybe Casey would like to have all those memories of you—"

"*I must to go!*" Leja shouts, jolting suddenly from her chair. "*I cannot listen this!*"

"Leja . . . but Joy is just—"

"I come tomorrow in the morning," she insists, marching out the door.

Joy does a double take. "What was *that*?"

"You know Leja . . . so emotional."

Joy nods.

But what we don't know is that Leja is headed back to the bungalow to report to Scott—huffing and puffing—her version of what just took place. Half an hour after she storms out of my room, Scott calls to tell me something so off-the-wall funny that he has to pause a few times midstory to laugh at his own words.

"So Leja just came home and she's got that face on, you know, like she's going to explode . . ." Scott begins.

"She was pretty upset when she left here," I confirm.

"And she says—*ha-ha*—in all seriousness, that—*ha-ha-ha*—Joy wants to help you die so she can marry me!"

"Oh my God . . ."

"Yeah. *Ha-ha-ha* . . ."

"What'd you say to her?"

"I laughed—which made her mad, of course. But it was the most ridiculous . . ."

"It's crazy!"

"I told her she's wrong, but she won't hear it. She feels she has to protect you . . ."

"From Joy? Give me a break!"

Joy hears her name and perks up. "What about me?"

"One sec . . . one sec . . ." I tell Scott I have to go, we'll talk later.

I bring my hands to my head. "You're not going to believe this, Joy, but Leja went back to the bungalow in an insane rage and told Scott that you are helping me die so you can marry him!"

Joy pauses before responding. She frowns deeply. "Wow."

"Scott laughed at her—really, he thinks it's so funny . . ."

"Hmm, yeah . . ." Joy ponders. "I guess we should expect nuttiness from her. But I have to say, this is hurtful—because I really feel like I've taken Leja under my wing every time I've been here. I've made a point of spending alone time with her, listening to her fears and trying to explain things in a way that helps her. I've praised her and said what a great friend she is to you. I even bought her a necklace . . . like this one." She tucks her pointer finger under the thin gold chain around her neck to show me—it says *Love* in tiny block letters. "Leja told me she liked it, so I got her one in DC and brought it with me on my next visit." She sighs wearily, throwing up her hands in bewilderment.

"Please, please—don't take her seriously. Scott and I have known Leja a long time. She can spin danger out of a sunny day at the beach. And once she gets an idea in her head . . ."

Joy springs from her chair. "Let's just move on, shall we?" She reaches for her toiletry bag while sliding her feet into slippers. "I think I'll wash up now, brush my teeth . . ."

I catch her hand as she shuffles past me toward the door. "Really,

Joy." I look up at her. "This is just too silly . . ." Her eyes are brimming with tears.

"Not to me," she says.

From: Joy Ceterra
Subject: The latest
Date: May 7, 2014 at 10:38 PM
To: Lauren Steale

Sweet Lauren, here is where I come out tonight.

The main thing we must stay focused on is Amy finding peace. Think of how much she has been through. It's not humane all these years. While we want her to go on for us and for Scott and Casey, we have to wish for what is best for Amy and only Amy.

So we have to try not to be sad. Try to think about Amy finding peace—if that comes from a new heart then we will be lucky too, but if it does not then I will accept it for her being at peace after 26 years of the most heroic fight we've ever witnessed.

I keep the strong faith that there will be a new heart but I wish for it only if it will give her the quality of life that she aches for.

Love you.

Joy

THAT NIGHT, WE manage to sleep only minutes at a time, not even half hours. But sometime around sunrise, my pacemaker firing quiets down and we are finally able to withdraw from the window and really settle in our beds. Sleep comes to both of us immediately and we give in to it, which means straying from our usual routine. Typically Joy spends some time emailing her office early in the morning and then wakes me at seven so I can get dressed and cleaned up before Dr. Kobashigawa arrives half an hour later. Today, though, for the first time in all of her mornings here, we are both still asleep at 7:10. We break our hospital ritual now because, it seems, this ritual has broken us. We can't keep doing what we've done all these weeks. Conditions have changed. As Joy said to me after two hours standing by the window last night, "This is a whole different ball game."

"Morning, morning . . ."

What? Dr. Kobashigawa . . . this early?

I open just one eye to make sure—yup, it's him.

Joy rouses drowsily and reaches down to check that her flannel pajama top is buttoned up.

The doctor remains standing, not taking a seat like he always does. "We have a donor for you," he says—just like that.

I sit up.

"We've been working on it all night. You're number one. It's yours."

"Hhhhhow . . . whaaa . . ." I press my fingertips against my cheeks to make sure I'm really here.

"It's an excellent heart from a thirteen-year-old girl."

I'm dazed, my voice full of wonder. "My first donor was thirteen too . . ."

"She is in great shape—an athlete, actually. And her parents donated all of her organs."

My eyes shift toward Joy with a shot of sorrow; the reality of this young death tempers my elation.

So many lives saved . . . but these poor, poor parents.

Dr. Kobashigawa continues, "She matches your antibody profile very well."

"Unbelievable," I whisper.

"But they still need to do the cross-match over there."

"Where?"

"A hospital in Nevada."

"So they have to . . . take all that blood and . . . helicopter it there, right?" I am pushing through the breathlessness now.

"No, actually, it's already there. We sent your blood just before you became a 1A."

I remember hearing about this from Emily a few weeks ago—how one particularly large blood draw I'd had was being divvied up and sent to various hospitals in nearby states where a donor heart might possibly wind up. My blood would be stored, she told me, and used for speedy cross-match if a donor was identified for me. It was supreme good luck that my blood had landed in storage at the hospital that now has a heart.

"Now," he continues, dropping his voice from kindly to cautioning and clear, "we won't know if this heart is viable for you until we get the results of the cross-match. I expect we will know by around four this afternoon."

"Okay, okay . . . so should I shower with the antimicrobial . . . ?"

"No, not yet. A lot can happen between now and surgery. A lot. So I suggest you enjoy the day, eat breakfast if you want—the surgery wouldn't happen until sometime this evening. Emily or I will be in touch."

"Wow, oh, wow . . ." My hand rises to cover my face; I'm looking through trembling fingers. "I can't believe . . . I really didn't think there would ever be a match for me. Six days left on my wall count, Dr. Kobashigawa. *Six.*"

His eyes sparkle as he smiles. "I told you to have faith."

"I couldn't . . . I am so sick and . . . everything seemed so impossible . . . I just . . ." A tear slips onto my cheek.

"I'm so pleased, Amy," he says, stepping toward me. I expect him to extend his hand for our customary parting shake, but no. This time, he holds out his arms. "Come here, darlin'," he says, and reaches down to hug me.

I lift my arms and wrap them around his white coat while tears stream silently down my face.

SCOTT AND I decide that we are going to keep this news mostly quiet. The exploding heart—and the plummeting of my spirits afterward—taught us a hard lesson. Scott calls Casey, I call my family, and when

Jody arrives in an hour or so, we will tell her everything, of course. But otherwise, for now, the excitement has to stay here in this room.

Meanwhile, an unfamiliar exhilaration is coursing through me. I feel myself brightening from head to toe. My knees quiver. My hands shake. My breath starts to quicken, and I turn my head to Joy for reassurance. "Whoa, help me out here. I don't want to whip myself into frenzy now, you know? Not sure my heart can take this much excitement."

"Got it!" She jumps from chair to bed and nuzzles up to me playfully. "Shhh . . . okay now, let's be a couple of *cool, cool* cats . . ."

"I do not like cats," Leja announces.

Joy shoots her a barbed look and whispers in my ear, "*Hold me back . . .*"

She's had it with Leja.

What happened between them last night has set Joy's mind against her, and even today's happy news doesn't douse the still-smoldering peeve. I didn't notice it until Leja just interjected with the anti-cat declaration, but now the tension is pervasive and uncomfortable. I feel bad for Joy. And this makes it impossible for me to share in Scott's laughing it off.

"I have to say something here—sorry, everyone . . ." I announce. "I want to get this out in the open and far away from this happy day, okay? Okay. What you said to Scott last night, Leja, was pretty darn silly . . . absurd, actually."

She purses her lips like she's just tasted lemon—*harrumph.*

I tsk-tsk at her, more playful than disapproving. As off base and extreme as her warning was to Scott last night, I understand the driving force behind it. Leja has long been my fierce protector, and I hers.

Scott takes over jovially, "*Re-diculous!*"

Leja straightens up proudly, putting on an air of righteousness. "Joy was taking notes to Amy, for what to do when she is dead. This to me is not a good friend!"

"Yes, it is, Leja . . . it *is!*" There is a lilt in my voice, but I mean to convince her. "The best friend is the one who knows you like you know yourself . . . and who loves you enough not to push her needs and her wants onto you."

She waves me off. "I do not agree. Sorry." Her voice is clipped. Final.

Scott grabs Leja around her waist and squeezes her into a tickle hug, "Leja, *Leja* . . . you are funny!"

The corners of her mouth turn up reluctantly.

"I am putting the matter aside," Joy says, "because it is totally ludicrous."

"And on a day like this . . ." I add, "we allow only good thoughts and kind words and . . ."

Dr. Kobashigawa appears in the doorway.

He strides into the room and stops short of handshake position. "Well—you're a nearly perfect match with your donor," he says. "I couldn't be more pleased with the cross-match—so here we go . . ."

A collective roar comes up. Joy jumps from her chair. Scott lurches toward me with both arms open, sweeping me into an embrace. Over his shoulder, I see Lachalle pop up behind Dr. K in the entryway vestibule, grinning delightedly. "We're going to need to take some blood now for the eculizumab treatment," the doctor continues, "and you'll have your first infusion in about an hour and then another one during surgery. After that, you'll shower"—Lachalle smiles even more gleefully and lifts the bottle of antimicrobial wash so I can see it—"and put on a gown, and I think you're scheduled to head into the OR sometime between around seven and eight tonight."

"This is really happening, then . . ." Scott says, bug-eyed.

"Oh, yes, this is happening," he confirms, shaking Scott's hand and then turning to me. "I'll see you sometime tomorrow—although I'm not sure you'll remember." I get a handshake too. Then Joy and Leja.

Lachalle moves aside to make room for him. "*Amyyyy!*" she cries. "You got your heart!"

IT'S EVENING AND my hospital room settles into a contemplative quiet. Jody is here now (Jack is away on business), along with Joy, Scott, and

Leja. Each of them has their own chair and their own private thoughts. There is no talk. After the swirl of medical activity—blood work, an antibody treatment, more blood work, chest X-ray, EKG, and my long, sudsy shower—the moment has arrived when the focus narrows and intensifies: in just a little while, a heart will be cut from my chest and a new one sewn into place.

On the other side of this marvel is its sheer enormity. A family has suffered an unfathomable loss and, without weeks or days or even hours to mourn, has risen up with mind-boggling beneficence that awes and humbles me now just as it has for decades. Heart transplant has its underside of medical shortcomings and travails, to be sure, but organ donation is one hundred percent beneficence and altruistic perfection.

I close my eyes for a moment and imagine the mother of the teenager whose heartbeat may soon become mine. A deluge of emotion floods my mind with longing: oh, how I wish I could reach out, right this second—person to person, mother to mother—and assure her that if I am lucky enough to survive this surgery, I will take the very best care of her child. For I have already watched over and nurtured one thirteen-year-old donor-heart girl, devoted every last bit of myself to protecting her from harm, doing all I can to keep her beating strong and free from heart transplant ills. And now I will do the same for this second lifesaving daughter-angel.

"Don't you worry—I've got this," I whisper under my breath. "You can count on me."

Lachalle comes in and I quickly wipe away tears, but she senses them anyway, nodding slowly and smiling. She hands me a clean gown—the first one I'm glad to put on here at Cedars. I slip off my sweatshirt but leave on my black cotton leggings. She warns me that they're not sterile and that the surgery team is going to make me take them off the minute I step into the operating room.

"Step in? Doesn't she get wheeled in?" Joy asks.

"No. Amy won't get any sedation until she's on the table, so she's just gonna walk on in there."

"I couldn't have done that two hours ago!" I chirp, and everyone chuckles. Just a couple of hours ago, they'd seen me go loopy after receiving the intravenous infusion of Benadryl that preceded my first eculizumab treatment (to prevent a reaction to my first dose). By that point, Scott had spread the good news broadly to friends and family; my cell phone rang again and again—and for the first time since arriving in California, I answered every call. Jill happened to call just as the Benadryl swept through my veins and set my lips into an uncontrollable quiver. She screeched into the phone, "I'm so *happy!*" but all I could say in return was a very shaky, garbled "I can't talk, Jill. I mean, I *really cannot talk!*" This made her laugh and laugh—just like old times.

"All right, then, Amy, here's the plan," Lachalle announces. "I'm going to go fetch your wheelchair now and set it in front of your door. It's almost eight, so I'll check if they're ready for you."

"Thanks," I say, looking up at her and then down at my hands. I've already taken off my wedding ring in preparation for surgery. It occurs to me just now that I might never put it on again.

Joy notices my reflective turn. "Let's give Amy and Scott a moment. But first . . ." She approaches the bed, and I stand up to face her. She tears up immediately. So do I. We have no words at first, just a squeeze of hands and a deep meeting of eyes that hold the history of the three months passed since we stood outside my bedroom door and talked of my grandmother and the impossibility of being saved by the comfort of company in the darkest of nights.

"We did it, Joy," I whisper now, confirming out loud what we already know: that I would not be here at the end of the great and terrible waiting list challenge if Joy had not been immersed in it with me since the beginning. We bring our noses together and shut our eyes tight.

Next it's Leja. I know I've got to be strong and confident for her—she's already shuddering with emotion. "I'm going to do great," I say, and we hug.

And hug. And hug. And hug.

Her embrace is more like a clutch. Leja wants me to have this surgery, of course, but she's frightened of its severity. "They're going to save my life now," I assure her.

"Okay . . . yes . . . okay," she says, weeping, "they will do."

I have to sit on the edge of the bed when she finally lets go.

"Ames," Jody says, grinning, extending her arms down toward me. "Love you. You got this. See you soon. And what can I say? I'm so, so happy for you—and Jackie boy is crazed that he's not here. But he'll be back tomorrow morning."

"Love you, Jody." She retreats to the far corner of the room with the other girls. I turn my head and find them in a group hug—arms resting atop shoulders, foreheads tipped against one another. The all-too-familiar cot stands upright in a folded position beside them; no one needs to sleep in it tonight. A background of streetlights glows outside the large window, illuminating an ecstatic huddle among women who, before two months ago, had never met.

So much about this moment strikes me as extraordinary.

An image comes to mind, and I close my eyes to try to preserve it— I'm in a jubilant embrace with Jody, Leja, Joy, Ann, Robin, Val, and the other girls, all of us silhouetted in the prism of a rainbow. Jill's violet runs into Lauren's blue that seeps into Jane's green and becomes my yellow . . . We share one another's light and color, transforming and transformed each by each and shimmering.

A shiver runs through me.

My gosh, look at us—some kind of magic . . .

I sway as Scott's weight sets down beside me on the edge of the bed. I grasp at the mattress and pop open my eyes into the moment. Directly in our line of vision is the wheelchair that Lachalle has placed in front of the open door. Scott takes my hand and brings it to his lips. "Come back to me, okay?" he says, welling with tears. "Just come back to me."

"I will, Scotty. I can do this—you know I can . . ." I lay my head on his shoulder.

Dimitri, the night nurse, appears in the doorway. Justin is off to-night. "You ready?" he asks.

"Yup."

Scott helps me up. I walk to the wheelchair. Joy, Leja, and Jody are in the hallway now; they stand beside me with forced smiles and wave.

Bye, Ames . . .

See you in the morning . . .

Justin sends you a smoochy-smoochy . . .

"Joy—get your mind out of the gutter!" I tease as Dimitri unlocks the wheels and gives the chair a push. Scott walks alongside me through the silent, empty hallway. Around the corner we go to the green door at the end of the next straightaway. It's just an ordinary entrance, not even a double door. I never knew it was the heart transplant operating room—until now.

Dimitri tells Scott, "I will push her through here and you can say good-bye before she goes into the OR."

"All right."

The door opens, and I roll into a dimly lit passageway. Just five or six feet inside, we come to a stop in front of a set of wide doors. "This is it," he says, locking the wheels in place.

A kind-faced woman in a blue surgical cap emerges at once. "Come on in, Amy. We're ready for ya." She reaches for my arm and guides me to standing. "Okay, quick kiss now," she says, cheerfully. "We're gonna get going."

I lift my face to Scott and we kiss—quick—just like she says.

And the next thing I know, I'm lying flat on the operating table in a bright white room. A swarm of nurses and doctors dart here and there around me, all of them friendly and chatty. They want to know if I'm warm enough, what kind of music I like, whether I mind the light that's just above my head. They pull off my black cotton pants.

I can't breathe . . .

As jolly as this scene is, I bring to it the very reason I am here, on this table, with my arms splayed way out to the side now, perpendicular to my body and secured on cushioned boards. My heart steals my breath. I'm going to get another one that will restore it.

"Can you put me out?" I ask abruptly, loud enough for all to hear. "I just want to be put out, please. Take me out of this body . . ."

A burn of anesthesia shoots through the needle in my forearm . . .

A rush of elation!

The most wonderful, enveloping sense of ease.

My last thought: *Thank you! Thank you so m—*

It's one a.m.

Scott, Leja, and Joy wait at the bungalow.

The surgeon took off for Nevada in a helicopter from Cedars's roof hours ago, promising to call Scott's cell once he returns with the donor heart. Another surgeon in the Cedars-Sinai OR has already opened my sternum to facilitate swift removal of my sick heart at the moment the healthy one arrives.

Meanwhile, conversation at the bungalow has given way to stifling silence. Scott sits alone, unfocused, in front of some late-late-night TV. Leja and Joy settle outside on the porch overlooking the little garden. Every hour or so, one of them calls Scott's cell just to make sure it's working. Growing concern pervades the atmosphere now: Why is this taking so long? They don't dare exchange last-ditch guesses.

Donor hearts can explode, you know . . .

Scott pushes himself up from the couch, lands his palms on either side of his head, and begins to pace. Joy glimpses him through the window and pleads with outstretched arms, "For the love of God—ring, damn cell phone . . ."

And then . . . a sound.

A whirring.

Louder and louder it drones, until it becomes a roar—a palpable, trembling force that seems to be rising over the back side of the bungalow.

Joy and Leja rush down the few steps onto the gravel path and look to the sky . . .

A helicopter!

Red and colossal and powerful—racing, racing toward the Cedars tower just two blocks down San Vicente.

"Scott! Scott!" He hurtles toward the screen door and through. "Look!"

All hands grasp—Scott to Joy to Leja.

The helicopter hovers above the landing strip and then slowly, slowly . . . sets down.

Scott's cell phone rings inside the bungalow.

"Ah!" He runs at once to answer it. "Hello!"

It's the surgeon.

"I'm back. The heart is perfect. We're going to get started . . ."

From: Scott Silverstein
Subject: Update
Date: May 9, 2014 at 2:27 PM
To: Jill Dawson, Ann Burrell, Lauren Steale, Valerie Yablon, Jane Keller, Robin Adelson, Jody Solomon

Just saw Amy in the ICU. She was starting to come out of sedation, and I think she was motioning for a writing pad, or maybe the waving of the hand was telling me to get out. Not quite sure, but I'm sticking with the writing pad story for now.

It's always a bit of a shock to see Amy after a major surgery. But this time I was really surprised and amazed. Her color is terrific. Her feet (which had been looking gray) are now a beautiful, healthy pink, as are her fingers and cheeks. Considering she's got a bunch of tubes connected to various parts of her body and about 8 drips going at the same time, she really looks fantastic.

All that said, I don't want to get ahead of myself, as this is still early in the process. Bleeding remains an issue, and she is taking a bevy of new drugs and huge doses of immunosuppressives, including some experimental ones that have only been used on a handful of heart transplant patients. So, we should expect some bumps in the road and unexpected turns. But so far so good and seeing her looking so well is truly tonic for the soul. Speak to you all soon.

From: Jill Dawson
Subject: Re: Update
Date: May 9, 2014 at 10:25 PM
To: Scott Silverstein

Scotty, this is so completely wonderful. I can't imagine how you're feeling because I can hardly contain myself. I know everything is still so precarious, but all of your updates about Amy's developments have been so encouraging. She IS a warrior and she will fight. I continue to be amazed by her spirit and strength.

Oh yeah, and you're not so bad either.

Love you both.

Xo

TWO MONTHS LATER

———

How to explain what has taken place in me?

How to quantify something that is beyond all reasonable expectation? I can't pin it down. I can't make sense of it.

It just shouldn't be this way.

I shouldn't be this way.

For the first time since I was twenty-five years old, I feel well.

I mean really well.

So well that I've been jogging three miles a day, just eight weeks after my surgery. And it's easy.

My body hums with such effortlessness I forget that it houses me; I'm not lugging it around and willing myself through its ills as I did for all those hard heart transplant decades.

How is this possible?

At my final clinic appointment before heading back to New York, Dr. Kobashigawa tells me, "What you put in is what you get out," meaning that all the jogging and gym workouts I banked right up until the time the vasculopathy grounded me have primed my muscles and organs to snap back quickly to strength.

"But I don't just feel strong . . . I actually feel well. I'm not nause-ated all the time, like I was with my first transplant. I don't feel ill and achy and weak. I don't have infections every ten days. I tell you, Dr. Ko-bashigawa, I feel so much better at fifty than I did at twenty-five—it's mind-boggling."

This makes him smile and pull his white coat across his middle. "Well then . . . enjoy!"

"But how can it be?"

He drops his chin, tugs his stethoscope from his neck, and tucks it into his front pocket—then pauses, smiling, shaking his head slowly.

Finally, he shrugs and tells me, again, to enjoy. "We want you to live your life," he says.

Live my life . . .

My transplant life.

As wonderfully well as I feel, and as high-flying as I am on grati-tude, I am no less aware of my medical reality. This second transplant carries an even more daunting threat to my heart's longevity. And the antibody treatments have put me at a higher risk of cancer and serious infection.

I'm not sure how to respond to Dr. K.

Even though I will return to Cedars in thirty days for a checkup, this still feels like a parting moment, and I'd like to speak the truth of it with him.

I sit up taller on the exam table now, taking in a deep breath for confidence. "I'm going to live this life, you can count on it," I begin. "But . . . well . . . there's no free lunch, right? That's what you said a few weeks ago when I got scared about all the side effects and risks of eculizumab—you reminded me that, living with a heart transplant, there's no free lunch . . ."

"Ah, Amy." He chuckles lightly, the corners of his eyes crinkling with kindness. "Yes, you pay for that lunch dearly, we both know it. But you—you've got a special brand of determination. I wouldn't put any limit on how far you'll go with this heart." He reaches his arms out to me, and I know to come in for a good-bye hug. "And of course, we're all here for you."

As I'm pressed against his white coat, an entirely new feeling sweeps me up and away to a place of contentment and peace I've never known in my transplant years: for once, my doctor and I understand each other.

In fact, I've experienced nothing but understanding from the entire Cedars heart transplant team, as I realized all at once when I left the hospital some seven weeks ago. The nurses and aides on the sixth floor gathered to say good-bye to me that day and, to my surprise, present me with a special gift. "We wanted to do something for the transplant patients as they set out on their new lives," the head nurse told me, speaking for the semicircle of staff around her. "We hoped to say something meaningful to them, so we created this." She handed me a navy blue T-shirt rolled up lengthwise and secured by a red ribbon.

I unraveled it.

On one side was an image of a chest X-ray printed directly onto the cotton, along with a message that read:

We are honored to be with you on this new journey.

—*The Nursing Team*

The other side of the shirt read:

Life may not be the party we hoped for,
    but while we are here we might as well dance.

It was the wisest, most honest orientation to heart transplant life that I'd ever seen: a striking acknowledgment that I—and all T-shirt recipients—would pay for our lunch, side by side with the wisdom for how we might make the most of our exceptionally fortunate seats at the table.

I knew right then: *I'm going to eat it up.*

The years of life ahead of me may not be long, but they will be different from those that came before, and better—not because my health challenges will be fewer or less serious, but because the truth of them is no longer a lonely one.

I held the shirt to my chest as if it were a salve and wept warm, salty tears.

LEAVING FOR NEW YORK

Breaking the stillness of the very early morning, Scott and I roll the last of our suitcases along the dew-misted gravel path and out the gate to a cab that's waiting on San Vicente. "I got this," he assures me, lifting the first duffle into the trunk. I turn back to say good-bye to the garden.

"Five months since I first saw you," I say to the greenery all around. "A whole season!" I'm standing in my favorite spot—directly in front of a speckled rock propped to its two-foot vertical stance by smaller rocks and plantings. It's meant to be a little fountain of sorts—there's a water pump behind it that produces a glistening stream along the contours from top to bottom—but the flow has been inconsistent lately. This morning, there's none at all. The rock is practically dry.

That's okay, it can stop now, I tell myself. *It knows I'm leaving.*

Just then, a hummingbird zooms by and lands on a tree branch to my right.

"Oh, hello, Miss Hummingbird. Coming to say good-bye?" I ask, admiring the iridescent green feathers on her underside. "Fly away, fly away now. I'm leaving too," I say. But she doesn't move at all, holding remarkably still.

Another one darts by me and lands on the same tree. And then another follows.

I've got my hand to my chest now. "Look at that—*three.*"

And now here's another, and another . . .

I continue counting as the hummingbirds keep speeding to this wiry, leafless tree—the only one in the garden that happens not to be thriving. Each bird lands on a bare branch that will give no nectar, and yet they all stay there.

Six . . . seven . . . eight . . . "Ah! Oh gosh!" Tears spring to my eyes now. *Nine . . . ten . . .*

I hold my breath in amazement.

All at once, they whir up and scatter in unison—out of sight in just seconds.

I turn my head away from the tree, and just when my eyes land upon the rock, a single bubble spills over the top and water begins to flow.

Scott spies me through the gate and rushes to my side. "Hey, are you all right?"

I don't realize that I'm sobbing.

"I'm fine . . . uh, I mean, I'm great—Scotty, the birds . . . the fountain . . ." I describe quickly what I've just witnessed. "That was incredible. I have to tell the girls . . ."

A few minutes later, I slide into the back of the cab and send a group email from my cell phone.

VAL CALLS ME early the next morning, bursting with interpretation. "Ten hummingbirds—you know what that was, don't you? That's nine of us women from the spreadsheet . . . and the girl who gave you her heart."

ACKNOWLEDGMENTS

When I say that this book would not have been possible without the support of many, I mean it in the deepest sense. The names that appear below refer not only to the people who helped me navigate the publication of *My Glory Was*, but also—and more essentially—those who figured prominently into my being alive to write the first word to the last.

I must begin, then, by noting the insufficiency of the word *acknowledgment* in titling this page. Still, I must give my gratitude a written go.

In no particular order, I would like to thank:

My parents, Arthur and Beverly, and my sister and brother-in-law, Jodie and Steve—whose loving care, endless understanding, and decades of intrepid visits to be by my side in hospitals in New York and California have been at the foundation of all I have been able to do and accomplish, including this book.

Dearest friends who were next up on the spreadsheet when the baton passing ceased (because a donor heart arrived)—Deirdre and Sue—as well as others who were rooting for me from afar with incessant hope and the most devoted prayers. The universe would not have been stormed so forcefully in my favor without all of you.

Lenny, Jack, Jon, and Gary—four treasured friends whose names did not appear on the spreadsheet of women, but whose wisdom and shining presence in my hospital room (and in my life) have been and continue to be the stuff of wonder.

The business associates who made it possible for Scott to work remotely from California for many months—the exceptionally supportive Brent, John, and Peggy.

The heart transplant team and support staff at Cedars-Sinai who have seen me through with kindness, empathy, and excellence— Angela Velleca, Emily Stimpson, Jenna Rush, Ellen Anifantis, Stephanie Kagimoto, Genevieve Harlocker, and all the esteemed rest, as well as the brilliant, endlessly compassionate cardiologists, many of whom have performed on me the most adept heart biopsies a gal could wish for—Drs. Kobashigawa, Patel, Chang, Moriguchi, Kittleson, Azarbal, Geft, Czer, Ramzy, and Hamilton.

My literary agent, Rebecca Gradinger—a glorious friend in her own right—who manages somehow to see publishing potential in every email I write and every vignette I retell. With a steady planting of two feet in my camp, Rebecca has illuminated for me time and again the big picture, the end goal, and the joys that are worth the writing toil that precedes them. It is because of her encouragement and the arm-in-arm sense of our venturing forward together that I dared take on the journey of this second book.

My Harper Wave editors: Karen Rinaldi, who bought this book in its earliest stages and imbued the whole project with enthusiasm and insight. Sarah Murphy, who dove into my pages with an extraordinarily keen eye and incisive mind to help me distill the soul of this story from its complexity. And Hannah Robinson, whose excitement brought spark and a youthful view from start to finish.

Stephen Koch, my wise literary beacon of can-do inspiration whose mere utterance of "Yes, and what's in the next chapter?" contained the magic to make me believe I could actually go forth and write it.

My fantastic Casey, who understands and shares along with me the love and angst of creativity, and the exhilaration and trepidation of facing the empty page. How wonderful it has been to learn and grow alongside my artist son throughout the writing of this book, and always.

And finally, my beloved Scott—the man and the love and the soul behind every bit of my strength, every ounce of perseverance in my writing and in facing my continuing health challenges, and every positive thought and excited sense of accomplishment that has come with each completed page of this book. I adore you and thank you, my love.

ABOUT THE AUTHOR

Amy Silverstein is the author of *Sick Girl*, which won a Books for a Better Life Award and was a finalist for the Border's Original Voices Award. She earned her Juris Doctor at New York University School of Law, has served on the Board of the United Network of Organ Sharing (UNOS), and is an active speaker and writer on women's health issues and patient advocacy. She lives in New York.